FROM ICU LESSONS TO
AI INNOVATION

OPPORTUNITIES IN HEALTHCARE

Redesigning our Medical Systems in the Age of AI, Prevention, and Courageous Leadership

Kwadwo Kyeremanteng

LUCKY BOOK PUBLISHING

LUCKY BOOK PUBLISHING

Published by Lucky Book Publishing: LuckyBookPublishing.com

The author does not dispense medical advice or prescribe the use of any technique as a form of treatment for physical, emotional or medical problems without the advice of a physician, either directly or indirectly. The intent of the author is only to offer information of a general true nature to help you in your quest for emotional, physical and spiritual well-being. In the event you use any of the information in this book for yourself, the author and the publisher assume no responsibility for your actions.

To request permissions, contact the publisher
at hello@luckybookpublishing.com.

For speaking opportunities and coaching inquiries, visit DrKwadwo.ca

Paperback ISBN: 978-1-998287-91-8
Hardcover ISBN: 978-1-998287-90-1
E-book ISBN: 978-1-998287-92-5

First edition, July 2026

Keywords: Healthcare Innovation; Healthcare Transformation; Healthcare Leadership; Artificial Intelligence in Healthcare; AI in Medicine; Future of Healthcare; Healthcare Reform; Healthcare Systems; Medical Leadership; Physician Leadership; Preventive Healthcare; Prevention Over Prescription; Lifestyle Medicine; Health Optimization; Longevity; Population Health; Healthcare Technology; Digital Health; Medical Innovation; Healthcare Management; Organizational Change; Courageous Leadership; Transformational Leadership; Physician Burnout; Healthcare Burnout; Patient Care Improvement; Healthcare Workforce; Staffing Shortages; Healthcare Costs; Hospital Management; Healthcare Policy; Community Health; Health System Redesign; Healthcare Entrepreneurship; Clinical Innovation; Leadership Lessons from the ICU; Healthcare Transformation Through Prevention, AI, and Courageous Leadership; Building Better Healthcare Systems; Prevention-Based Healthcare; Healthcare Executive Leadership; Future of Medicine; Resilience and Health; Patient-Centered Care; Sustainable Healthcare; Health System Innovation.

Disclaimer

A Note on the Stories in This Book.

As a physician, protecting patient confidentiality is one of my highest responsibilities. While many of the stories in this book are inspired by real experiences, they have been intentionally altered to protect privacy. In many cases, they are composites that blend elements from multiple patients, and some are fictionalized examples created to illustrate broader principles. No individual patient is being described.

My hope is to share the lessons these experiences have taught me while honoring the trust that patients and their families place in their healthcare team.

MY GIFT TO YOU

I am so glad you're here!

As my Gift to you, get FREE Access to resources and other bonus content by scanning the QR Code below or visiting drkwadwo.ca

"When we align our values, think integratively,
focus on what truly matters, and take courageous action,
we create flow."

– Dr. Kwadwo Kyeremanteng

Contents

Preface

Why Now?

Much to the quiet concern of my wife, who is likely discovering this confession as she reads these very words, there's another book. Yes, Cathy, it happened again.

We've explored leadership.

We've explored prevention.

Now it's time to talk about transformation, specifically, how we can repair a healthcare system that's no longer serving the people who depend on it.

This book isn't about blame. It's about possibility. Because, despite the frustration and fatigue so many of us feel, I still believe we have everything we need to create a system that truly works, for patients, for healthcare workers, and for society as a whole.

When I wrote *Unapologetic Leadership*, my goal was to challenge how we think about courage and authenticity, how leaders show up when the stakes are high. When I wrote *Prevention Over Prescription*, I wanted to give people the tools to take ownership of their health through nutrition, movement, sleep, stress, and community.

This book is the bridge between the two. Because leadership without wellbeing collapses. And prevention without system change will always fall short.

Over the past several years, I've seen the best and the worst of our healthcare system. I've seen compassion that moves you to tears, teamwork that feels miraculous, and clinicians who give more of themselves than anyone should ever be asked to give. But I've also seen burnout, inefficiency, and frustration: people working harder than ever but often feeling like it's never enough.

I've seen the cracks widening:

- Patients waiting months for basic imaging
- Families unable to find a primary-care provider
- Emergency rooms overflowing into hallways
- Clinicians burning out faster than we can replace them
- Mental health supports out of reach for those who need them most
- A system buckling under administrative complexity and outdated processes

We all know something is wrong. We also know the system is full of brilliant, committed people who want to do better but who are trapped in structures that make it nearly impossible. And yet, despite all the frustration, I remain optimistic. Amid all the challenges, I see signs of renewal.

We have the tools to turn things around:

- Artificial intelligence to predict deterioration before it happens
- Digital systems to streamline referrals, diagnostics, and follow-up care
- Community-based programs that promote prevention and connection
- Innovative leaders ready to think differently and act boldly

The ingredients for transformation already exist:

We have the technology.

We have the data.

We have innovative models working in pockets across the country.

We have passionate, creative people ready to lead.

We have communities hungry for change.

What we are missing is alignment: a unifying strategy, a clear direction, and the belief that meaningful change is possible.

That is what this book aims to offer.

A Blueprint for Reform

This is not another policy textbook.It's not a partisan argument. It's not an academic analysis for experts only.

This is a **call to action** rooted in:

- lived clinical experience
- frontline stories
- system-level research
- leadership science
- behavioural design
- innovation
- prevention

At the heart of this book is a simple question:

What if we designed healthcare around humanity instead of bureaucracy?

To answer that, we'll explore:

- stories from the ICU and beyond

- inefficiencies that create harm and waste
- the crisis in primary care
- the mental health emergency
- opportunities in prevention
- the role of technology and AI
- how public-private partnerships can strengthen, not weaken, universal healthcare
- and the leadership frameworks needed to bring it all together

The organizing principle behind it all is the Pareto Principle: the 80/20 rule. Twenty percent of interventions account for most of the outcomes. Our goal is to identify those few high-impact, high-leverage changes that can transform the system **without waiting for a revolution**.

From Individual Agency to Collective Action

Prevention Over Prescription gave individuals agency over their health. This book expands that agency to the level of hospitals, clinics, communities, and the system as a whole.

It's about:

- scaling prevention
- turning compassion into culture

- using technology wisely
- modernizing processes
- empowering clinicians
- strengthening primary care
- reducing wait times
- building a system that works for the next generation

We cannot wait for someone else to fix healthcare. We are the system: the clinicians, patients, administrators, innovators, and families who experience it daily hold the solutions we need.

If this book does its job, it will remind us that reform is not only possible. It is already happening in small but powerful ways. We simply need to amplify what works, align around shared values, and take decisive action.

The time for hope backed by execution is now.

Let's begin.

Introduction
A Lesson From the ICU

When I was training, I cared for a young man (let's call him *Chad)* who had been in a devastating car accident that left him paralyzed and dependent on a ventilator. Through perseverance and excellent care, he was finally making progress. With the help of our respiratory therapists and physiotherapists, he was slowly regaining his ability to breathe on his own.

Then came a long weekend. Due to cost-saving measures, physiotherapy coverage was cut back. By Monday morning, Chad had relapsed. He was back on the ventilator. Weeks of progress were erased, not because of medicine, but because of management.

That moment stayed with me. It revealed something that has haunted our system for decades: we too often cut where we should invest. The very people and programs that move patients forward, the physiotherapists, the discharge planners, the social workers, are the first to go when budgets tighten. That short-sightedness planted a seed.

From the ICU to a Movement: Why Prevention Is the Most Important Leadership Challenge of Our Time

When you work in the ICU, you see life in its sharpest contrast.

You see triumph: a patient walking out after weeks on a ventilator.

You see heartbreak: a family saying goodbye far sooner than they ever imagined.

You see resilience: fear, courage, and human fragility layered on top of each other.

But you also see something else, something harder to accept:

Most of the suffering that ends up in the ICU is preventable.

I've cared for middle-aged men in kidney failure from decades of unaddressed hypertension. I've seen women with metabolic disease who never had a chance at proper guidance or support. I've held the hands of elderly patients who deteriorated because they waited 16-18 hours in an overwhelmed emergency department. I've treated young people pushed to the brink by sleep deprivation, stress, isolation, and burnout.

Each case is unique, but the patterns are unmistakable:

- Poor sleep

- Chronic stress
- Ultra-processed diets
- Sedentary living
- Isolation and loneliness
- Limited access to primary care
- A reactive health system, not a preventative one

This isn't a moral failing.

This is a **systems failing**.

We have brilliant clinicians, compassionate professionals, and world-class technology, yet the structure they work within is not built to prevent disease. It is built to *treat it once it becomes catastrophic.*

A Call to Do Better

Frustrated but hopeful, I pursued a Master's in Health Administration and founded the *Resource Optimization Network* to study how we could improve care while reducing waste.

We published nearly a hundred papers. We proved that smarter use of resources could improve outcomes and save money.

But the truth? Little changed.

Policy alone wasn't moving the needle. Data wasn't enough. The system wasn't short on information. It was short on courage, creativity, and connection.

So, I pivoted. Through *Prevention Over Prescription*, the podcast, and a growing digital community, we began empowering individuals to take control of their health. And it worked. People started reversing chronic conditions, improving their metabolic health, and rediscovering hope.

But while individuals were healing, the system around them continued to deteriorate. Our hospitals became bottlenecks. Our healthcare workers burned out. And far too many people fell through the cracks before ever reaching care. Over time, I began to ask questions that made me deeply uncomfortable:

What if most of what we call "healthcare" is actually sick care?

What if prevention isn't just a lifestyle issue, but the leadership issue of our generation?

And what if the most powerful tools to change health are not medical procedures, but purpose, alignment, community, and behavior?

Those questions pushed me out of the ICU in a new way. Not to leave it, but to understand how to keep more people from ever needing it.

The Birth of PRESS

In working with patients, executives, athletes, and frontline clinicians, I noticed something striking:

People didn't need more complex guidance. They needed clarity. Health wasn't being lost because people were lazy or undisciplined. It was being lost because the *fundamentals*, purpose, sleep, nutrition, movement, relationships, were never prioritized, taught, or supported.

Out of this came **PRESS**: **Purpose, Restoration, Eating, Strength, Social.** These are the fundamentals that determine energy, resilience, metabolic health, mental health, and longevity.

Five pillars.

High impact.

Evidence-based.

Accessible.

Human.

PRESS became the operating system I used with individuals and teams wanting to take control of their health in simple, sustainable ways. But something else was happening in parallel. As I spoke to leaders, hospital CEOs, policy makers, corporate executives, medical departments, I recognized a second barrier:

People knew *what* to change. They didn't know **how** to change systems. That required a different framework.

The Birth of VIPA

I realized that if we wanted healthcare to feel human again — if we wanted organizations to reduce burnout, increase alignment, and actually execute on prevention — they needed a model for culture, collaboration, and forward motion.

That model became **VIPA**:

- Values - your compass
- Integrative Thinking - seeing beyond silos
- Pareto + Psychological Safety - focusing on what matters most while empowering people to speak and innovate
- Action - the courage to move, iterate, and learn

VIPA is how movements start. It's how we built the **Black Medical Collective** in 60 days with no budget, a movement that has now helped more than 15 young Black leaders gain acceptance to medical school. It's how we created **Lionheart Innovation**, bringing clinicians, researchers, and entrepreneurs together to accelerate discovery and solve real health challenges. It's how organizations, departments, and leaders can create *flow*: alignment between purpose, people, and process.

Together, **PRESS and VIPA are the two operating systems of this book.**

PRESS transforms individual health.

VIPA transforms systems.

One without the other is incomplete. This book brings them together, so individuals can thrive, teams can align, and leaders can create change that lasts.

How to Read This Book

- Part I lays the groundwork for prevention and identifies foundational areas for action.
- Part II identifies opportunities to support comprehensive healthcare in ways that can be integrated into our culture and systems.
- Part III looks to the potential of technological and systemic developments and maps future potential for growth.

Every chapter includes stories, science, practical tools, and reflection prompts.

This is not a book about willpower. It's a book about systems, the ones that shape our health, and the ones we can build to change it.

Let's begin.

Part I
The Foundations of Prevention

Chapter 1

The VIPA Framework: How Leaders Create Flow

"When we align our values, think integratively, focus on what truly matters, and take courageous action, we create flow."

- Dr. Kwadwo Kyeremanteng

Healthcare is overflowing with brilliance, yet too often, brilliance is trapped in silos. Clinicians, administrators, and innovators are all rowing hard but not always in the same direction. The result? Bureaucracy instead of collaboration, burnout instead of purpose, and incremental tweaks instead of transformation. If we want a system that feels human again, a system that prevents rather than merely reacts, we need **flow**. Flow happens when purpose, people, and process move in rhythm.

The VIPA Framework is a blueprint for creating alignment and forward motion in clinics, hospitals, communities, and even personal health journeys. It's not theoretical;

it's lived. It's how we move from chaos to clarity, from burnout to belief. The same principles that transformed a mentorship program can transform medicine itself.

Values anchor us in humanity amid AI and automation.

Integrative Thinking helps us blend digital precision with human empathy.

Pareto focus reminds us to direct resources toward prevention, not paperwork.

Action keeps the mission alive when bureaucracy slows progress.

Flow happens when these four forces align. That's how we'll move from sick-care to healthcare, from reaction to prevention. Healthcare has plenty of intelligence. What it lacks is *alignment*.

> People do not burn out because they work hard. They burn out because their effort has no momentum.

Flow happens when people understand the mission, feel psychologically safe, collaborate across disciplines, and move with shared intention.

VIPA is a blueprint for creating that flow.

V – VALUES: The Compass That Guides Every Decision

Our values define the culture of care, whether we lead with empathy, fairness, and courage or fall into complacency and hierarchy. Values are not slogans. They are the behaviors you will defend even when it is inconvenient.

When values are clear:

- Teams trust each other.
- Decisions become aligned.
- Leaders act with courage instead of fear.
- Culture becomes consistent, not personality-dependent.

In medicine, values transform "one more shift" into service, advocacy, and meaning.

They give clinicians permission to say:

"This is not acceptable."

"This does not align with the care we want to give."

"This is not who we are."

Values anchor change.

I – INTEGRATIVE THINKING: Dissolving Silos to Create Better Solutions

One of the most transformative ideas in my life came from Roger Martin, world-renowned strategist and former Dean of the Rotman School. I had the privilege of sitting down with him on my podcast to talk about **Integrative Thinking**, and that conversation, no exaggeration, changed everything for me.

Roger explained that the best innovators don't choose between opposing models; they *integrate* them to create something better. Integrative Thinking is about synthesis over separation: holding two ideas in tension and building a superior third option.

Imagine you're creating a new film festival. You study **Cannes**, exclusive, elegant, globally prestigious, and **Toronto (TIFF)**, inclusive, accessible, audience-driven. An either/or mindset says you must copy one. An *integrative* mindset asks:

> "What if we take Cannes's polish and Toronto's accessibility and design a festival that's both world-class *and* community-powered?"

That's integrative thinking in action. It's the same in healthcare. When designing a clinic or wellness center, instead of choosing between a high-tech model and a community-based model, ask:

> "What if we merged cutting-edge AI diagnostics with the warmth of human coaching?"

Integrative Thinkers don't choose between competing models. They synthesize them and create something better. The future of healthcare requires synthesis, not silos. True reform happens when clinicians, technologists, policymakers, and patients co-create solutions.

Healthcare desperately needs this mindset:

- Virtual care and in-person care
- Tech-enabled diagnostics and human coaching
- Public health and personalized prevention
- Innovation and equity
- Efficiency and empathy

When we dissolve silos, possibilities expand. The future of healthcare isn't built by any single profession. It's built at the intersections, where clinicians, technologists, policymakers, entrepreneurs, and communities co-create more humane solutions. Integrative thinking makes that possible.

P – PARETO + PSYCHOLOGICAL SAFETY: Focus on What Matters + Build the Culture to Support It

The Pareto Principle tells us that 20% of actions lead to 80% of results. But in healthcare, Pareto only works if people feel safe enough to speak openly. Psychological safety is not softness. It is the foundation of high performance.

When teams feel safe:

- They raise concerns early
- They innovate freely
- They challenge outdated practices
- They share information instead of protecting it

We focus on what matters most, high-impact priorities, while cultivating safety for people to challenge, question, and innovate without fear. Together, Pareto + Safety create high-leverage cultures where the most important work gets done by teams that trust each other.

A – ACTION: Imperfect, Bold, Forward

You can have values, brilliant ideas, and smart focus, but nothing changes until someone moves. Progress demands motion. Ideas are only as powerful as the action they inspire. Action is not reckless. Action is iterative. You start, learn, adjust, refine, and evolve.

Every movement in healthcare, from quality improvement to prevention programs to new clinics, succeeds because someone decided:

“We are not waiting for permission.”

VIPA turns clarity into motion. It turns motion into momentum, and momentum into change.

VIPA in Real Life: The Black Medical Collective

After the murder of George Floyd, I felt a responsibility deeper than commentary. I looked around the ICU, hospitals, conferences and realized how often I was the only Black physician in the room.

Representation was not symbolic. It was structural. It shaped trust, access, and opportunity. Out of that conviction, we built the **Black Medical Collective** using VIPA:

Values

Equity, representation, courage.

Integrative Thinking

Mentorship + visibility + real opportunities: mock interviews, research placements, volunteer roles, networking, storytelling.

Pareto + Safety

A focus on the activities that matter most for admissions; a safe space to speak honestly about race, bias, belonging, and confidence.

Action

We launched in 60 days with zero budget. Today, more than 15 mentees have been accepted into medical school, one with four offers, another with over $100,000 in scholarships.

Values → Integration → Focus → Action.

This is flow. This is VIPA.

Worksheet: Putting VIPA in Motion

1. Define Your Challenge: What systemic issue or personal goal do you want to tackle?
2. Map Your Values: List 3–5 guiding principles that will anchor your approach.
3. Integrate Perspectives: Who can you bring together from different disciplines, communities, or lived experiences?
4. Identify Your 20 Percent: Which specific actions will drive the majority of results?
5. Commit to Action: Write one concrete step + timeline. Execute, reflect, iterate.

Final Thoughts

The VIPA Framework isn't just a leadership model. It's a philosophy for transformation. When we lead with **Values**, think **Integratively**, focus through **Pareto and Psychological Safety**, and take bold **Action**, we create the conditions for flow in our organizations, our communities, and our own lives. Progress in healthcare, and in life, doesn't begin with perfection. It begins with purpose in motion.

Reflection

1. **Values:** Which three words define the culture you want to build? How visible are they in your daily behavior?
2. **Integrative Thinking:** Where are you trapped in either/or decisions? How can you combine the best of both worlds?
3. **Pareto/Safety:** What 20 percent of actions would yield 80 percent of the improvement? How will you create safety for honest dialogue?
4. **Action:** What imperfect step can you take this week to move forward?

Write your answers. Revisit them often. VIPA is a practice, not a checklist.

Key Takeaways

- The root of healthcare dysfunction is misalignment.
- The solution won't be built by any single profession.
- Real change happens through imperfect but decisive action.

Chapter 2

Costs and Improving Efficiency: Why Smarter Care Saves Lives and Saves the System

---

"The greatest waste in healthcare is not money. It is preventable suffering."

- Dr. Kwadwo Kyeremanteng

If you spend enough time in an ICU, you begin to see the patterns, not just the clinical ones, but the systemic ones. You see how patients arrive in crisis, how earlier conversations could have prevented suffering, how fragmented care leads to unnecessary investigations, and how millions of dollars quietly evaporate through inefficiency.

And you begin to recognize an uncomfortable truth:

Healthcare is not just strained; it's financially hemorrhaging. And most of that hemorrhage is preventable.

As an ICU physician, I deal with the downstream consequences. I see the end stage: patients at their most fragile. But after two decades of practicing medicine, leading teams, researching system performance, and living the reality of hospital gridlock, I am convinced that improving efficiency is just as critical as improving access. This chapter is about the cost of inefficiency, financially, clinically, ethically, and how we can do better.

The Hard Economics of Inactivity and Chronic Disease

Let's start with one of the biggest elephants in the room: lifestyle-driven chronic disease.

Physical inactivity alone costs Canada's healthcare system **$3.9 billion every year** in *avoidable* healthcare expenditures. Let that sink in. These are not costs we're obligated to incur. These are preventable.

Researchers estimate that just a **15% increase in physical activity** among Canadians could save **$1 billion annually** across:

- Reduced chronic disease
- Fewer hospitalizations
- Lower medication use
- Less absenteeism in the workforce
- Decreased disability

A billion dollars saved simply by helping people walk more, move more, lift weights, and build healthier habits.Prevention is not a "nice to have." It's a powerful economic strategy. But prevention is chronically underfunded. We pour money into acute care, hospitals, surgeries, ICUs, but neglect the upstream factors that determine who ends up sick in the first place.

Critical Illness: The Most Expensive Care We Deliver

Few people realize how expensive critical care truly is. In Canada, **1% of our entire GDP** is spent on treating critically ill patients. That's billions of dollars every year. And ICU care is just the tip of the iceberg. Every admission comes with downstream costs:

- Rehab
- Long-term care
- Home care
- Disability support
- Lost income
- Caregiver burnout
- Mental health strain
- Follow-up appointments
- Hospital readmissions

One ICU admission often triggers months or years of resource use. This is why prevention (metabolic health, physical activity, nutrition, sleep, connection) has such massive potential. When someone ends up in my unit, the system is already losing the battle. We can save lives, yes. But the toll, on the patient, the family, and the system, is enormous.

And so much of it is preventable.

A 90-Year-Old Transfer That Should Never Have Happened

She was 90 years old. Living in a nursing home. Advanced dementia. Congestive heart failure. Stage 3 kidney disease. Frailty that was obvious the moment you looked at her legs and arms: muscle wasted away, skin thin as paper. The kind of patient whose goals of care should be meticulously documented and easily accessible to every provider involved in her life.

But that day, no one had access to her wishes.

In Canada, every institution uses a different electronic medical record. The nursing home chart doesn't sync with the hospital chart. The hospital chart doesn't sync with the outpatient clinic. And paramedics often receive nothing more than a photocopied transfer letter, if that.

So, when she aspirated during dinner, something not uncommon for patients with advanced dementia, she became hypoxic. Her vitals looked concerning. The staff, erring on the side of caution, did what they are trained to do: transfer to the ED.

No goals-of-care form. No accessible documentation. No provincial-level EMR. Just a frail 90-year-old woman sent into the machinery of acute care.

In the emergency department there was bloodwork, a chest X-ray, broad-spectrum antibiotics, fluids, monitoring, and discussions with consultants. When her breathing worsened, the default response was escalation. In the absence of documented wishes, she was intubated.

I met her the next morning in the ICU, sedated, ventilated, wrists restrained to prevent self-extubation, a woman who could no longer tell us what she wanted, but who *had* told her family many times: “I don’t want aggressive care near the end of my life.”

Her daughter, devastated, said to me, “She would have never wanted this.”

Total cost of care for that admission?

$15,000–$20,000, easily.

But the financial cost paled in comparison to the human cost.

The suffering.

The indignity.

The emotional trauma for the family.

The burden on an overstretched ICU.

The bed that could have gone to someone who needed it.

All because we didn't have a unified EMR or clear documentation. This case, and thousands like it every year, is the definition of avoidable inefficiency. Not cutting corners. Not denying care. Just **knowing what matters to the patient**.

This is why efficiency is not just financial stewardship, but compassion, respect of human dignity, and good medicine.

The $10,000 Transfer for a Simple UTI

Now, consider a very different scenario.

A patient in a small rural hospital develops a urinary tract infection. They present with fever, discomfort, and mild dehydration. Their blood pressure is stable. Their lactate is normal. Their sepsis score is low. A straightforward case.

But the local hospital is short-staffed that day. Perhaps the on-call physician is newer and uncomfortable managing potential sepsis. Maybe the lab turnaround times are slow. Perhaps the hospital has no rapid response team or has limited access to specialists. Or maybe it's simply that the culture in that institution is: *When in doubt, transfer.*

So, the decision is made to send the patient to a tertiary care hospital.

Here's what that sets in motion:

- Paramedic activation
- EMS transport
- ED triage
- Repeat bloodwork ("just to be safe")
- Repeat imaging ("because outside imaging doesn't integrate into our EMR")
- Another round of antibiotics
- Monitoring
- Mandatory reassessment before discharge

Total cost: **$8,000–$12,000** for a condition that could have been managed locally with:

- IV antibiotics
- Fluids
- A sepsis protocol
- Clear criteria for escalation
- A remote physician hotline or virtual support
- Better integration of diagnostics

These cases happen **every single day** across Canada. Not because clinicians don't care. Not because they're incapable. But because the system is designed in a way that encourages inefficiency:

- No unified EMR
- No cross-site communication
- No shared protocols
- No virtual mentorship
- No incentives, financial or otherwise, to treat locally
- No redundancy built into small hospitals

Every avoidable transfer contributes to:

- Congested tertiary EDs
- Backlogged hospitals

- Longer wait times
- Increased hallway medicine
- Patient frustration
- Burnout among staff
- Higher costs

And the saddest part? It's preventable.

Efficiency Is Not About Cuts. It's About Smarter Care

There's a misconception that talking about efficiency means talking about cutting services or rationing resources. But that's not what efficiency is.

Efficiency means:

- Doing the right investigations, not the most.
- Using the right medications, not the most expensive.
- Treating patients in the right location, home, community, or hospital, depending on need.
- Preventing avoidable deterioration.
- Communicating clearly across providers.
- Respecting patient goals.

- Avoiding duplication.
- Using technology intelligently.
- Implementing evidence-based care pathways.
- Prioritizing interventions with the highest impact.

That is not rationing. That is responsible medicine. And it's what patients want.

The Choosing Wisely Campaign: A Bright Spot in Canadian Healthcare

One of the most effective strategies we've seen in the last decade is the **Choosing Wisely** campaign. It has encouraged clinicians to ask:

"Do I really need this test?"

"Will this change management?"

"Is this medication necessary?"

"Is this intervention aligned with the patient's goals?"

Choosing Wisely has helped reduce:

- Unnecessary imaging
- Routine daily labs
- Duplicate testing
- Low-value screenings

- Inappropriate antibiotics
- Non-beneficial interventions

It's a cost-efficiency program disguised as a quality initiative. And that is why it works. Patients benefit. Clinicians benefit. The system benefits.

Choosing Wisely proves that efficiency does not mean sacrificing care. It means improving care.

Why a Unified EMR Is Essential

Let me be blunt: Canada's fragmented electronic medical record landscape is a threat to patient safety and a colossal driver of waste.

We have:

- Nursing homes on one system
- Family doctors on another
- Hospitals on five others
- Walk-in clinics on something totally different
- EMS with paper printouts

This results in:

- Duplicate imaging
- Duplicate labs

- Missed diagnoses
- Medication errors
- Inappropriate transfers
- Misaligned goals of care
- Increased length of stay

A province-wide unified EMR would:

- Surface goals of care instantly
- Provide a single source of truth
- Reduce redundant testing
- Improve discharge planning
- Support community providers
- Facilitate telemedicine
- Enable predictive analytics
- Save millions

It's expensive up front, yes. But the return on investment is massive. Alberta and Quebec have already moved in this direction. Ontario, British Columbia, and others need to follow. This is one of the most important efficiency plays we can make.

The Cost of Inefficiency Shows Up Everywhere

Let's zoom out for a moment.

Inefficiency contributes to:

1. Longer Wait Times

When tertiary hospitals are clogged with avoidable transfers, waitlists grow. Elective surgeries get delayed. Emergency rooms get backed up. Hallway medicine becomes the norm.

2. Burnout Among Healthcare Workers

When the system wastes resources, human beings make up the difference. Clinicians work harder, not smarter. Exhaustion follows.

3. Worse Outcomes

Delays cause disease progression. Transfers cause instability. Poor communication leads to inappropriate treatment.

4. Financial Waste

Every $10,000 transfer, every unnecessary ICU day, every duplicate test compounds across millions of patients.

5. Mistrust in the System

Patients see the chaos, the delays, the confusion, and lose confidence.

Efficiency isn't optional. It's survival.

Prevention: The Ultimate Efficiency Strategy

When people remain metabolically healthy, physically active, and connected to their communities, they stay out of hospitals.

They avoid:

- ICU admissions
- Surgeries
- Diabetes complications
- Heart attacks
- Strokes
- Joint replacements
- Long-term medications
- Specialist visits

> Prevention is the single most underutilized cost-saving tool in Canadian healthcare.

Walking, strength training, adequate protein, sleep, managing stress, reducing processed foods: these are not lifestyle hacks. They are system-level interventions.

This is why I'm so passionate about the PRESS framework, and why I believe preventive coaching should be part of universal care. Prevention isn't just good for individuals. It is the backbone of an efficient, sustainable system.

Public–Private Partnerships: Another Path to Efficiency

This topic gets politicized quickly, but the truth is simple:

Public dollars can go further when used smartly.

Specialty surgical centers, private clinics performing publicly funded procedures, diagnostic hubs: these can dramatically increase throughput. The Shouldice Clinic is a perfect example: They consistently perform hernia surgeries faster, safer, and more efficiently than most hospitals.

This isn't ideology. This is math. If we want shorter waitlists, more throughput, and better outcomes, we need to expand capacity, not just within hospitals but alongside them.

This is a core theme of this book: **Innovation + efficiency = better care.**

Discharge Teams & Rehab: Small Cost, Huge ROI

There are few things more efficient than high-functioning physiotherapists, occupational therapists, social workers, and discharge planners who work proactively.

Early mobilization, equipment planning, home-care setup, family education: all of this gets patients home sooner and prevents readmissions.

A great discharge team:

- Reduces length of stay
- Reduces deconditioning
- Reduces delirium
- Increases functional independence
- Prevents hospital readmissions
- Improves quality of life
- Saves money

Cutting these positions is one of the most short-sighted decisions hospitals make. Investing in them is one of the smartest.

Efficiency Is Care

When we talk about efficiency, some people fear that we're cutting corners or replacing judgment with cost. But that couldn't be further from the truth.

Efficiency means:

- Knowing patient goals
- Avoiding unnecessary suffering
- Reducing harm
- Providing dignified care
- Helping people stay in their community
- Reducing delays
- Supporting clinicians
- Using resources responsibly so that everyone who needs care can receive it

Efficiency is compassion.

Efficiency is respect.

Efficiency is sustainability.

Efficiency is the future of healthcare.

Where We Go From Here

We must shift from a reactive, crisis-driven model to one that is thoughtful, proactive, and value-oriented. That means:

- Investing in prevention
- Expanding community capacity
- Implementing unified EMRs
- Reducing unnecessary transfers
- Empowering local hospitals
- Supporting clinicians with protocols and virtual backup
- Doubling down on discharge planning
- Using Choosing Wisely principles daily
- Reinforcing primary care
- Aligning incentives to reward value, not volume
- Treating patients where they are, whenever possible

Because the reality is simple: **The money we save through efficiency becomes the money we reinvest in innovation, prevention, staffing, and patient experience.** Efficiency is how we build a system Canadians can trust again.

Final Thoughts

Every dollar wasted through inefficiency is a dollar we cannot spend on prevention, mental health, innovation, primary care, or surgical throughput. Every unnecessary ICU admission is a missed opportunity to have prevented suffering. Every avoidable transfer is a symptom of a fragmented system. Every duplication of care reflects our failure to coordinate.

But the reverse is also true:

- Every efficient decision honors patient values.
- Every avoided transfer frees up space for someone who truly needs it.
- Every unified EMR reduces harm.
- Every step toward prevention builds a healthier population.
- Every discharge done well creates dignity and autonomy for a patient.

Efficiency is one of the greatest untapped levers for reforming healthcare, and it's one of the most compassionate. If we want a healthcare system that works, not just for today, but for decades to come, then improving efficiency is not optional. It is essential and urgent. And it begins now.

Reflection

1. Where in our current healthcare system are we spending the most money without meaningfully improving patient outcomes?
2. What is one area of waste that, if addressed, could reduce suffering for patients and stress for healthcare workers?

Key Takeaways

- Efficiency is compassionate, and the root of it is not about cutting resources.
- Inefficiency causes burnout and financial waste.
- Prevention is the most powerful cost-saving strategy.

Chapter 3

Primary Care: The Cornerstone of a Healthy System

"If you want a strong healthcare system, start at its foundation."

- Dr. Kwadwo Kyeremanteng

George was a 56-year-old mechanic and father of two who hadn't had a family doctor for almost five years after his clinic closed. He was healthy, active, and stubbornly independent. One spring weekend, he noticed a painful swelling on his arm, likely a simple infection. He thought about the ER but couldn't stomach waiting half a day in a crowded hallway, so he tried to manage it himself. By the time he finally came to our ICU, the infection had spread to his bloodstream. Despite every effort, we couldn't reverse the damage.

His death was preventable. If George had access to a primary-care team, a nurse practitioner, virtual physician, or even a pharmacist trained to triage, he'd likely be alive today. That's the cost of a broken foundation. And sadly, his story is not unique. Across the country, countless "Georges" fall through the cracks: minor infections that become sepsis, undiagnosed hypertension that becomes stroke, small lumps that become late-stage cancer, all because access was denied or delayed.

Primary care is the heartbeat of any healthcare system. It's where prevention happens, where relationships are built, and where early warning signs are caught before they become life-threatening. Yet, across Canada, and especially in many underserved regions, nearly one in five people have **no primary-care provider at all.** The consequences are devastating, and increasingly visible in our emergency rooms, hallways, and ICUs.

Why Primary Care Matters

Primary care isn't just about writing prescriptions or managing coughs and colds. It's about **prevention, coordination, and trust.** Family doctors and nurse practitioners are often the catalysts for screening, vaccination, and lifestyle change. They're the reason a patient gets that colonoscopy that finds a precancerous polyp early, or finally starts managing their blood pressure, or feels supported enough to start walking again after depression.

> When we neglect primary care, we neglect prevention, and the cost is measured in both dollars and lives.

Dr. Jane Philpott, in *Health for All: A Doctor's Prescription for a Healthier Canada*, reminds us that universal access to a "primary-care home" isn't a luxury; it's the organizing principle of a humane system. Jurisdictions that guarantee every citizen a longitudinal relationship with a primary-care team consistently show **better outcomes, higher satisfaction, and lower cost per capita.** She argues that we must build "teams not silos," family physicians, nurses, social workers, dietitians, and community health navigators working together under one roof. It's not more medicine; it's better coordination.

The Challenge

The shortage of family doctors has reached a critical point. In provinces across Canada, hundreds of thousands, millions, of patients are "orphaned," reliant on emergency departments for what should be basic family-medicine care. Meanwhile, fewer new physicians are choosing family medicine as a career.

Why? Because the economics and structures no longer make sense. Family physicians carry overwhelming administrative loads, struggle with outdated fee codes, and often earn less than specialists, despite being the backbone of the system. The result: fewer doctors enter the field, workloads increase for those who remain, burnout rises, and access worsens.

Dr. Philpott has argued that we must **"re-professionalize family medicine"**: restore its status, modernize its pay structures, and integrate it into team-based, salaried, or blended-funding models that emphasize continuity over throughput. She's right. If we truly believe in *Prevention Over Prescription*, this is where the work begins.

Reimagining Primary Care: What We Can Do Now and Tomorrow

1. Value and Support Our Family Doctors

If we claim that prevention and community health are priorities, our compensation models must reflect that. Family doctors should be among the most valued professionals in healthcare, financially, emotionally, and structurally.

That means:

- Fair remuneration that recognizes complexity and time spent with patients, not just procedures.

- Administrative and digital support to reduce paperwork.
- Team-based funding models that reward prevention, follow-up, and patient continuity, not just visits.

Investing here isn't charity; it's smart economics. Every dollar spent on robust primary care saves multiple dollars downstream in avoided ER visits and hospitalizations.

2. Leverage Virtual Care to Close the Gap

During the pandemic, **Renfrew County** built one of the most innovative models: a *Virtual Triage and Assessment Centre* connecting residents without a family doctor to physicians anywhere in Ontario. A patient in Renfrew could be cared for by a doctor in Timmins; labs and imaging were done locally; follow-ups happened online. It wasn't perfect, but it worked, and it should become **standard infrastructure**, not a pandemic relic.

To scale it:

- Properly remunerate virtual visits.
- Build interoperable systems that let labs, imaging, and notes flow seamlessly.
- Pair virtual care with local pharmacists, nurses, or community clinics for in-person support.

- Recognize virtual attachment as legitimate continuity for patients without in-person access.

Virtual primary care can bridge the gap for millions if we treat it as essential public infrastructure.

3. Adopt National Licensure for Physicians

There's no clinical reason I, as an intensivist in Ontario, can't treat a patient in Alberta or Manitoba virtually. Medicine doesn't change at provincial borders, but our licensing rules do.

A national licensure system would:

- Enable cross-provincial virtual care.
- Allow redeployment of clinicians to shortage areas.
- Support equitable access in rural and remote communities.

It's complex, but solvable. We've tackled harder things: organ transplantation, genome mapping, pandemic vaccines. We can fix this too.

4. Empower Nurse Practitioners and Physician Assistants

Expanding access doesn't mean diluting quality. NPs and PAs are highly trained and can manage most primary-care issues, escalate when necessary, and build continuity with patients. This team-based model strengthens, not replaces, family doctors, freeing them to focus on complex and preventive care. A layered, collaborative approach should be our norm.

5. Streamline Pathways for International Medical Graduates

Thousands of skilled physicians trained abroad remain sidelined by opaque, inconsistent licensure processes. Some drive taxis or work lab jobs while towns go without doctors.

We need competency-based assessments, bridge programs, and provisional licenses that integrate qualified clinicians quickly and safely. If someone is capable and motivated to serve, there must be a place for them. We can't claim to value access while keeping qualified hands idle.

6. Integrate Prevention, Data, and Social Determinants

Primary-care reform isn't just about volume, but vision. Clinics should be designed around prevention: cancer screening, metabolic assessments, mental-health check-ins, and early intervention.

Imagine every annual visit including:

- A metabolic-health score and preventive dashboard.
- Nutrition and exercise counselling linked to local programs.
- AI-powered reminders for vaccines and screenings.
- Automatic referral to social supports when housing, food, or loneliness issues arise.

Prevention doesn't require new technology; it requires **integration and intention**. Technology should free clinicians to connect, not click.

7. Create Community-Based Primary-Care Hubs

Dr. Philpott advocates for "primary-care homes," interdisciplinary hubs where care, diagnostics, and prevention live side-by-side. Imagine community spaces where you can see your family doctor, join a nutrition workshop, get bloodwork, and attend a wellness class under one roof. These hubs already exist in pockets across Canada, from Quebec's CLSCs to B.C.'s Urgent and Primary Care Centres, and they work. They embody what prevention looks like in practice: local, relational, team-driven.

8. The 80/20 of Primary-Care Reform

Applying Pareto's principle, a small set of interventions will yield most of the benefit:

1. Value and fund primary care properly.
2. Expand virtual care and national licensure.
3. Deploy NPs, PAs, and international grads.
4. Integrate prevention, technology, and social supports.

These are the 20 percent of levers that will solve 80 percent of the crisis.

Final Thoughts

Every story like George's reminds me: reform isn't theoretical; it's urgent. We can build a system where everyone has a family-care home, where prevention is rewarded, and where no one has to choose between waiting eighteen hours in an ER or risking their life.

That vision starts with **Values**, respecting and supporting those who deliver this essential care. It continues with **Integrative Thinking**, linking technology, virtual care, and new provider models. It thrives on **Psychological Safety**, empowering clinicians to innovate without fear. And it ends with **Action.**

Let's make family medicine a career young physicians aspire to, not avoid. Let's let technology bridge distance rather than create bureaucracy. Let's ensure that every Canadian, urban, rural, or remote, has access to the kind of relationship that saves lives long before they reach the ICU.

Because the cornerstone of a healthy system isn't just access. It's the belief that **every person deserves it, and that we have the courage and imagination to build it.**

Reflection

1. What would healthcare look like if every person had timely access to a trusted primary-care team before crisis occurred?
2. Where are people in your community most likely to fall through the cracks, and what would it take to catch them earlier?

Key Takeaways

- The family doctor shortage is a policy failure.
- Primary care is an economic necessity and a cornerstone of prevention.
- Virtual care is an underused resource that can drastically improve care access.

Chapter 4
Advanced Care Planning: Honouring Wishes, Avoiding Suffering, and Doing What's Right

---

"The way your loved one dies is never forgotten."

- Dr. Kwadwo Kyeremanteng

She was 93 years old. Frail. Living in a long-term care home. Multiple comorbidities: advanced dementia, congestive heart failure, chronic aspiration, severe frailty, and mobility issues that made every movement an effort. Anyone who cared for her knew she was at the final chapter of her life. What they didn't know, because it was never documented, was what she actually wanted when her time came.

One evening, she aspirated while eating. Her oxygen plummeted. Staff called 911. Paramedics arrived. And in the absence of clear advanced directives, the default took over. Full code. Full resuscitation. Full intervention.

She was rushed to the emergency department, intubated, sedated, and admitted to the ICU. Two days later, her family, finally reached by phone, told us softly and tearfully, "She never wanted any of this."

She had apparently told them countless times that she didn't want aggressive life-sustaining measures. She wanted comfort. She wanted peace. She wanted dignity. But the moment passed. The decisions were made. The default happened. And none of it aligned with her values.

This story is tragic, but unfortunately, it's typical. According to the Canadian Institute for Health Information (CIHI), a significant proportion of older adults receive aggressive end-of-life care that does not match their preferences, especially when no advance care plan has been documented. In the United States, similar patterns exist: studies published in JAMA and the New England Journal of Medicine show that many patients at the end of life undergo ICU admissions, mechanical ventilation, and resuscitation despite previously expressing a desire to avoid aggressive care.

Mrs. D received care she would never have chosen, care that caused suffering, consumed enormous resources, and left her family heartbroken. And it all could have been avoided with one simple intervention:

A conversation.

The Human Cost of Silence: What Happens When We Don't Talk

Avoiding discussions about end-of-life wishes doesn't just create confusion. It creates suffering. And not just for the patient, but for everyone involved.

1. Patients Receive Care They Do Not Want

Multiple studies have shown that a large percentage of elderly, frail, or cognitively impaired patients receive invasive treatments inconsistent with their values when advance care planning is missing. Research from the Institute of Medicine (in their landmark report "Dying in America") found that many patients nearing the end of life receive burdensome care that fails to improve survival, function, or comfort.

Patients often undergo:

- Intubation
- CPR (which in frail older adults often causes fractures, internal injuries, and almost never restores meaningful life)
- Ventilation and sedation
- Repeated hospital transfers
- Painful procedures with little benefit

These are not small interventions; they're life-altering. And the absence of planning leaves the system to choose for the patient. And the system chooses aggressive.

2. Families Are Thrust Into Impossible Decisions

When families don't know what their loved one would want, they carry a burden that lasts a lifetime. I've seen guilt, regret, and trauma in the eyes of sons, daughters, and spouses forced to decide about life support for someone they love. Research from the University of Toronto and Harvard shows that family members making decisions without guidance experience significantly higher rates of depression, anxiety, and complicated grief, even years later.

But when a patient's wishes are known, families experience:

- Less stress
- Less guilt
- A feeling of honouring their loved one
- Peace in the grieving process

As someone who has lost both parents, I say this from a deeply personal place: How your loved one dies stays with you forever. And clarity is one of the greatest gifts they can leave behind.

3. The Healthcare System Bears Enormous Costs

Aggressive end-of-life care is not only misaligned with patient preferences. It is also extremely expensive. CIHI reports that care in the last year of life represents nearly one quarter of total healthcare spending in Canada. ICU care is particularly costly: an ICU bed can cost $3,000–$5,000 per day, and end-of-life ICU admissions frequently last one to three weeks.

The "Choosing Wisely" campaigns across multiple countries emphasize that much of this care is low-value and does not improve survival or quality of life. In fact, studies published in JAMA Internal Medicine show that early palliative conversations reduce ICU utilization, improve quality of life, and lower costs by up to 36%, without affecting mortality.

But the cost is secondary to the human impact. What we really save with advance care planning is suffering.

Advanced Care Planning: What It Actually Means

There's a misconception that advance care planning (ACP) is simply signing a form or checking a box. It's far more than that. Advance care planning is a process, an ongoing, values-based conversation that ensures medical decisions align with what matters most to the patient.

ACP helps answer questions like:

- What does quality of life mean to you?
- What level of disability or dependence would be acceptable to you?
- What are you afraid of?
- What would you want if you couldn't speak for yourself?
- What wouldn't you want tolerated (ventilators, CPR, feeding tubes, repeated hospital transfers)?
- Who do you trust to make decisions for you?

This is not about choosing death. This is about choosing dignity. And it gives clinicians permission to align care with the patient's values, not the system's defaults.

The Role of Clinicians: Guiding, Recommending, Not Just Asking

One of the biggest failures of our current approach is that we ask families and patients: "What do you want us to do?"

This is the wrong question.

Families aren't medical experts. They are grieving, overwhelmed, and often in shock. They shouldn't be asked to decide between intubation, CPR, or vasopressors at 3 a.m. in the emergency department. Instead, clinicians should ask:

"What mattered most to your loved one when they were well?"

"How did they feel about independence, quality of life, and comfort?"

"Did they ever talk about what they would want at the end of life?"

Then the clinician should make a clear recommendation based on those values and the clinical reality. Health systems that have implemented structured ACP (such as Kaiser Permanente, Alberta Health Services' Goals of Care program, and Australia's national advance care directive framework) show that when clinicians lead with recommendations, rather than endless options, patients and families experience far better outcomes, clarity, and peace.

The evidence is clear:

- Early goals-of-care discussions improve patient satisfaction
- Advance directives reduce ICU utilization
- Palliative care improves symptoms, mood, and even survival in certain cancers
- Families experience less depression, anxiety, and PTSD
- Clinicians experience less moral distress

This is not soft medicine. This is good medicine.

Why People Avoid These Conversations

Despite overwhelming evidence of the benefits, ACP remains underutilized. Studies suggest that only 30% of adults have any form of documented end-of-life plan. Why?

1. Cultural Avoidance of Death

Death feels uncomfortable. We avoid discussing it. But ironically, avoiding the conversation makes dying far more difficult.

2. Clinician Discomfort

Medical training often emphasizes saving lives, not guiding peaceful deaths. Many clinicians feel ill-equipped to initiate these discussions, even though research shows most patients want them.

Harvard's "Conversation Project" found that while 92% of people believe ACP is important, only 32% have had the conversation.

3. Fear of Causing Distress

Some worry that initiating these conversations will upset patients. But multiple studies show the opposite: patients feel relief, not distress, when asked.

4. Misunderstanding of Palliative Care

Many equate "palliative" with "giving up." But palliative care is simply the pursuit of comfort, alignment, and quality of life, and many patients receive it while continuing active treatment.

The Call to Action: How We Fix This

To prevent more stories like Mrs. D's, we need a cultural shift in how we approach end-of-life care.

1. Make ACP a Standard Part of Primary Care

Every annual check-up for patients over 65 should include an ACP conversation. This is standard in parts of the U.K. and Australia and has been shown to reduce unwanted ICU admissions.

2. Implement Structured Goals-of-Care Systems Nationwide

Alberta's "Goals of Care Designation" is a national model: a standardized, provincially recognized form documenting patient wishes in plain language. Research from the province shows this system reduced unwanted transfers from nursing homes and improved clinician confidence.

3. Train Clinicians in Values-Based Conversations

Communication training works. Programs like VitalTalk, Ariadne Labs' Serious Illness Conversations, and the Canadian national framework all show improved patient satisfaction and reduced unwanted interventions.

4. Encourage Families to Talk Before Illness Occurs

The best ACP discussions happen around kitchen tables, not hospital beds.

5. Normalize Revisiting Decisions

Values change. Health changes. ACP should be reviewed every few years and after major life events.

A Personal Reflection: Why This Matters to Me

Losing both of my parents changed how I view life and how I view death. I will never forget:

- the moments that felt aligned
- the moments that were chaotic
- the clarity we had
- the confusion we wished we didn't

As a son, I understand the emotional weight. As a physician, I see the consequences every day. The truth is:

> A good death is one of the most important, sacred gifts in healthcare.

And it doesn't happen by accident. It happens by preparation.

What a "Good Death" Actually Looks Like (According to Research)

Studies from the University of British Columbia, Stanford, and Harvard have identified key elements of a good death:

- Pain and symptoms are managed
- Preferences are known and honoured
- Unwanted medical interventions are avoided
- The person is surrounded by those they love
- No unnecessary transfers or hospitalizations
- Spiritual or cultural needs are respected
- A sense of dignity and control is preserved

These aren't luxuries. These are achievable outcomes when planning happens early.

The Financial Lens: Why ACP Is Also Smart Policy

Though this chapter focuses primarily on dignity, quality of life, and human suffering, the economics matter too. Health systems with robust ACP programs (U.S. Veterans Affairs, Kaiser Permanente, and several Australian states):

- reduce ICU use by 25–40% in the last month of life
- reduce hospitalizations by 20–30%
- dramatically increase patient and family satisfaction
- reduce moral distress among healthcare workers

CIHI reports that end-of-life costs could be reduced substantially if palliative approaches were initiated earlier. ACP is not an expense. It is a cost saver. But more importantly, it is a human saver.

A Framework for Clinicians: How to Have the Conversation

Here is a simple, evidence-based approach used by programs like VitalTalk:

1. Ask Permission

"Would it be okay if we talked a bit about your health and what matters most to you?"

2. Explore Values

“What brings your life meaning?”

“What would you consider a good day?”

“What are your biggest fears about your health?”

3. Align Clinical Reality

Share prognosis honestly but compassionately.

4. Recommend

“Given everything you’ve shared, here’s what I would suggest...”

5. Document and Communicate

Document clearly. Share with family. Update regularly.

A Pearl of Wisdom From Critical Care

After caring for thousands of critically ill patients, here is the truth: Death is not the worst outcome. Suffering without purpose is. A death misaligned with a person’s values is.

And we can prevent that.

Final Thoughts

Advanced care planning is one of the most important acts in healthcare. It is not paperwork. It is not bureaucratic. It is not pessimistic.

It is:

- a roadmap
- a safeguard
- a gift
- an act of clarity and love
- a promise to honour someone's story, not overwrite it with the system's defaults

For patients, it means dignity.

For families, it means peace.

For clinicians, it means alignment and clarity.

For society, it means compassion and sustainability.

As someone who has lost both parents, who has stood at thousands of bedsides in the ICU, who has seen suffering that could have been avoided, this chapter is not theoretical for me. It's deeply personal.

We owe it to our loved ones, to our patients, to ourselves. Let's have the conversations. Let's normalize them. Let's teach them. Let's honour people's wishes. Because the way someone dies matters. And it will never, ever be forgotten.

Reflection

1. Have you had a conversation with the people you love about what matters most if illness or crisis occurs?
2. How can healthcare teams make advanced care planning feel less like giving up and more like honouring dignity?

Key Takeaways

- Getting end-of-life care right is sacred work.
- Lack of advance care planning can lead to direct harm and aggressive treatment.
- Families' burdens are significantly lessened when wishes are documented clearly.

Part II

Cultural Change and Reclaiming Health

Chapter 5
The PRESS Method: Prevention at Scale

"Small changes done consistently can change your health, your community, and even the healthcare system."

- Dr. Kwadwo Kyeremanteng

As many of you know from my second book, *Prevention Over Prescription*, I've spent years trying to move healthcare upstream, to help people take control before illness takes control of them. What excites me now is that people finally *want* this.

There's a cultural shift happening. Everywhere I go, from hospitals to corporate boardrooms to high-school gyms, I see people searching for a better way to live. They don't just want to survive; they want to *thrive*. They want energy, strength, focus, and connection. They want to be proactive about their health.

For decades, healthcare has been reactionary. We wait for crisis. We wait for disease. But prevention is gaining momentum because people are realizing that their daily choices, what they eat, how they move, how they sleep, who they surround themselves with, determine the quality of their years long before disease ever appears on a chart.

That's the world I want to help build: one where prevention is the default, not the afterthought.

Karen's Story

Karen was an executive in her late forties, smart, high-performing, and completely depleted. She was 25 pounds overweight, running on caffeine and adrenaline, and living squarely in the "sandwich generation": teenagers on one side, aging parents on the other. Sleep was poor, nutrition was inconsistent, and exercise had become a distant memory.

She came to us not for vanity but for survival. "I'm functioning," she said, "but I'm fading."

We started small. We identified her priorities and narrowed them down using the 80/20 rule: what two levers would move the needle most? The answer was simple: protein and sleep.

We focused on hitting her protein target every day and creating a digital sunset: no phone after 9 p.m., lights dimmed, magnesium before bed. The result? Within four months, she lost 20 pounds, reversed her pre-diabetes, and felt like herself again. Her energy soared, her confidence returned, and her leadership flourished. Her kids noticed; her team noticed; *she* noticed.

But here's what struck me most: Karen's transformation didn't just benefit her. It reduced her future healthcare burden. Multiply that by thousands of people, and prevention becomes not just personal. It becomes *policy*.

Why PRESS

To bring prevention to scale, I needed a simple, repeatable structure, something you could teach in schools, prescribe in clinics, and apply in workplaces. That's how the **PRESS Method** was born:

P - Purpose

R - Restoration (sleep + stress)

E - Eating (nutrition + metabolism)

S - Strength (movement + resilience)

S - Social Connection

PRESS is more than an acronym; it's a lifestyle operating system. It helps people *press* toward health rather than being pulled toward illness. It's built on two guiding philosophies:

1. The Pareto Principle (80/20 Rule): Focus on the 20 percent of habits that create 80 percent of the results.
2. Progress Over Perfection: Health isn't about doing everything; it's about doing something that matters every day.

When you combine focus with consistency, you create momentum, and momentum changes lives.

Purpose: The North Star

Purpose gives health meaning. Without a "why," every "how" eventually fades.

In the ICU, I've watched patients fight through impossible odds when they had something, or someone, to fight for. Conversely, I've seen others give up when that purpose felt lost.

Purpose doesn't have to be grand. It could be *being around to walk your daughter down the aisle*, *coaching your son's hockey team*, or *leading your company with energy instead of exhaustion*. Karen's "why" was her family. For others, it's community service, faith, or simply wanting to feel proud in their own skin again. Whatever it is, anchor to it. When you know your "why," health becomes non-negotiable.

Restoration: Sleep and Stress

Restoration is the most underrated performance enhancer on the planet. Sleep is when your body repairs, your hormones rebalance, and your brain consolidates memory. Stress, meanwhile, is the silent accelerator of disease. Modern life has convinced us that burnout is a badge of honor. It's not. It's a warning sign.

Here's what I tell patients and executives alike:

- **Defend your bedtime.** Go to bed and wake up at the same time daily.
- **Put your phone to bed before you.** Blue light suppresses melatonin and spikes cortisol.
- **Breathe.** The *physiological sigh*, two short inhales, one long exhale, can drop your stress in seconds.
- **Protect morning light.** Ten minutes of sunlight in the morning sets your circadian rhythm for the night.

Restoration is not laziness; it's leadership. You can't pour from an empty cup.

Eating: Fuel, Not Friction

Nutrition is often where people overcomplicate and under-execute. The PRESS approach is simple:

1. Prioritize Protein. Aim for 0.7–1 gram per pound of ideal body weight.
2. Reduce Ultra-Processed Foods. They're designed for addiction, not nutrition.
3. Eat Real Food First. Whole foods beat supplements every time.
4. Stay Hydrated. Water and electrolytes trump sugary drinks.

I call protein *the 80/20 of the 80/20* because it changes everything: satiety, muscle retention, metabolism, and even mood. When people double their protein and cut processed foods, almost every metabolic marker improves. Energy rises. Cravings fall. Weight stabilizes.

Food can be medicine or poison. Choose medicine.

Strength: Building Your Body Armor

Muscle is not optional; it's protection. Strength training preserves independence, improves insulin sensitivity, and supports bone health. It is, quite literally, a life-saving habit. You don't need a gym. You just need gravity and commitment.

- **Lift 2–3 times per week.** Focus on compound movements, e.g., squats, push-ups, deadlifts.

- **Add "exercise snacks."** Ten squats between meetings, a plank while the coffee brews.
- **Walk daily.** 7,000 steps is enough to transform metabolic health.

I once cared for a man in his seventies who survived cardiac arrest because he was strong. Within days, he was walking, while still on a ventilator. That's what strength buys you: resilience. As we age, muscle becomes our most valuable currency. Build it while you can.

Social Connection: The Overlooked Medicine

Loneliness is now recognized as a public-health crisis. Studies equate its mortality risk to smoking 15 cigarettes a day. Connection, on the other hand, is deeply healing. It lowers inflammation, boosts immune function, and protects against depression.

Social connection doesn't happen by accident.
It's cultivated.

- Text the friend you've been "meaning to call."
- Schedule walking meetings instead of coffee meetings.
- Volunteer or join a community group.

Humans heal in community, not in isolation. Connection is medicine.

PRESS in Action: Shaping the Next Generation

Imagine bringing PRESS into our schools.

Kids today move less, sit more, and spend hours scrolling instead of exploring. Mental-health concerns and obesity are climbing. But it doesn't have to be this way.

A **PRESS Challenge** in schools could look like this:

1. **Assess.** Students rate themselves 1–5 in each PRESS pillar.
2. **Choose.** The class selects one focus area per month.
3. **Act.** They commit to small, measurable goals: 8,000 steps a day, 7 hours of sleep, 5 home-cooked meals per week.
4. **Reflect.** They journal progress and celebrate wins together.

This approach not only teaches health literacy, but builds teamwork, accountability, and empathy. It empowers kids to see health as something they *create*, not something that happens to them. Imagine the impact if every child graduated high school knowing how to cook a meal, manage stress, lift safely, and cultivate community. That's real health education.

PRESS for Our Elders

The same framework revitalizes our aging population.

Frailty is one of the strongest predictors of ICU admission and mortality. Yet it's reversible.

For seniors, PRESS could look like:

- **Purpose:** mentoring youth or volunteering.
- **Restoration:** consistent sleep and daily relaxation practices.
- **Eating:** prioritizing 100 grams of protein per day to prevent muscle loss.
- **Strength:** resistance bands twice weekly.
- **Social:** weekly group meals or walking clubs.

I've seen elderly patients regain independence simply by addressing those five levers. Prevention isn't just for the young. It's the difference between living long and living *well*.

PRESS in Workplaces: Prevention as Culture

Organizations thrive when their people are healthy. Absenteeism, burnout, and chronic disease cost billions annually, but more importantly, they cost joy.

Integrating PRESS into corporate wellness can be transformational:

- **Purpose:** Align work with mission and values.
- **Restoration:** Encourage "digital sunsets" and true lunch breaks.
- **Eating:** Provide real-food options, not just muffins and coffee.
- **Strength:** Incentivize walking meetings and office step challenges.
- **Social:** Build belonging through mentorship and shared wins.

Healthy people build healthy companies.

The Future: Peptides, GLP-1s, and Lifestyle Prescriptions

We're entering a new frontier of medicine where biology and technology converge. GLP-1s, peptide therapy, and personalized nutrition are reshaping metabolic health.

I'm optimistic. But the danger is believing medication alone can replace lifestyle. It can't. My vision is that every prescription will eventually come with a **Lifestyle Order**:

- Protein target
- Resistance routine
- Sleep plan
- Stress-reduction protocol
- Social connection commitment

Imagine a world where you're prescribed both a medication *and* a personalized PRESS Plan. One treats symptoms; the other treats the system. We're already seeing early signs: clinics pairing GLP-1s with coaching, peptide programs combined with strength training, and digital apps tracking nutrition and recovery. The future of healthcare will be *hybrid*: pharmacology + press = lasting change.

The Economics of Prevention

If we zoom out, the numbers are staggering. Every chronic disease prevented saves tens of thousands in lifetime healthcare costs. One avoided ICU stay can save $50,000 to $100,000. Multiply that by the millions living with preventable disease, and the case for prevention becomes undeniable.

Prevention isn't just good for people; it's good for budgets, businesses, and governments.

Worksheet: Design Your PRESS Plan

Area	Score (1-5)	One Action This Week	Accountability Partner
Purpose			
Restoration			
Eating			
Strength			
Social Connection			

Final Thoughts

The PRESS Method is more than a framework. It's a philosophy. It's a reminder that health is built, not bestowed. If we can help people rediscover their purpose, restore their energy, eat real food, build strength, and stay connected, we'll not only extend life but expand what it means to live.

When prevention becomes culture, hospitals quiet down, families thrive, and communities flourish. This is how we shift from a system that reacts to disease to one that builds health. This is how we press forward. Together.

Reflection

Find out your PRESS score:

1. Purpose: Why do you want to be healthy? Who benefits?
2. Restoration: How consistent is your sleep routine?
3. Eating: Are you hitting your protein and whole-food goals?
4. Strength: How often do you train or move intentionally?
5. Social Connection: Who energizes you, and how often do you connect?

Pick **one or two** areas to focus on this month. Create a 30-day mini-challenge. Track your progress weekly and reflect on how you feel.

Key Takeaways

- Prevention scales when it's simple.
- PRESS translates prevention into daily practice.
- When adopted widely in homes, schools, and workplaces, PRESS can reshape population health.

Chapter 6
Health Promotion by Design & Nudging: Making the Healthy Choice the Easy Choice

---

"When we design for health, we stop asking people to swim upstream alone."

- Dr. Kwadwo Kyeremanteng

A few summers ago, my family and I were walking through Paris on a crisp spring morning. As usual, we were on the hunt for a café, but along the way, we entered a park that changed how I think about health forever.

This wasn't just a park. It was a movement ecosystem. Joggers circled the pathways. Parents cycled past with their kids in tow. Seniors were doing tai chi in the shade. And then we saw it: an outdoor gym. Simple pull-up bars. Parallel bars. Stretching areas. No membership. No walls. No barriers.

And like any active family, we jumped right in. The boys challenged each other to pull-ups. My wife joined a Parisian stretching on the mat. I started doing dips beside an older gentleman with perfect form. We weren't "working out." We were simply responding to the environment. That moment hit me hard: This wasn't motivation. It was design. Health was built into the architecture of the city. Movement wasn't an appointment; it was a way of being.

That morning with my family became the blueprint for this chapter. If Canada wants better health outcomes, less chronic disease, more vitality, stronger communities, we need to stop relying on individual willpower and start redesigning the environments we live in.

Why Design Matters More Than Intention

People don't rise to the level of their goals; they fall to the level of their environment.[1]

Paris made movement effortless. Canada makes it optional.

Research shows that walkable cities dramatically reduce disease and extend lifespan.[2-5] Even simple daily steps reduce mortality by up to 50%, with most benefits occurring between 7,000–10,000 steps per day.[6-7]

TABLE 1 – Daily Steps & All-Cause Mortality

(Kraus et al. 2021; Paluch et al. 2022)

Steps/day	Mortality Risk	Evidence
<5,000	Highest risk	Sedentary = metabolic syndrome ↑
5,000–7,000	↓ 40–50%	Major reduction in mortality
7,000–10,000	↓ 50–70%	Optimal range
>10,000	Plateau	Diminishing returns

The Paris park didn't tell us to exercise; it invited us. That's what Canada needs to replicate.

Design Principle #1: Make Movement Unavoidable

Walkability, bike lanes, and accessible fitness equipment are not luxuries. They are public-health infrastructure.

The evidence is overwhelming:

- Walkable cities reduce obesity, diabetes, and cardiovascular disease.[8]
- Active transportation improves mental health and lowers inflammation.[9]
- Outdoor gyms increase spontaneous strength training and community use.[10]

TABLE 2 – Built-Environment Features & Health Outcomes

Feature	Health Impact	Evidence
Sidewalk networks	↑ steps; ↓ obesity	Sallis et al. (2012)
Protected bike lanes	↑ cycling; ↓ injuries	WHO (2016)
Outdoor fitness stations	↑ community movement	Chow et al. (2016)
Mixed-use planning	↑ movement & social connection	Giles-Corti et al. (2016)

A Canadian city designed like that Paris park would produce healthier citizens by default, not because of willpower, but because of architecture.

Design Principle #2: Healthy Food Needs Healthy Architecture

Our food environment is engineered to promote overeating. Ultra-processed foods (UPFs) now make up more than 50% of calories in many households. They dramatically increase the risk of obesity, diabetes, depression, and early death.[11-13]

TABLE 3 – Health Risks from Ultra-Processed Foods

Health Outcome	↑ Risk from UPFs	Evidence
Obesity	+50–60%	Monteiro et al.
Type 2 Diabetes	+59%	Public Health Nutrition
Depression	+20–25%	Meta-analysis
Hypertension	+35%	Monteiro et al.
Mortality	+62%	JAMA Int Med

We need environments that make whole foods the easy choice:

- Whole-food kiosks in public buildings
- "Protein-first" sections in cafeterias
- Labelling that highlights minimally processed foods
- Reduced-cost produce through government partnerships

The Paris park didn't rely on self-discipline. It relied on design. Our food system must follow the same principle.

Design Principle #3: Workplaces as Movement Ecosystems

What struck me in Paris was how inclusive the outdoor gym was. Seniors. Adults. Teens. Kids. Locals. Tourists. Everyone could join. Canadian workplaces could become the same:

- Resistance-training hubs in office buildings
- Walking meeting policies
- Step-count incentives through insurance
- PRESS coaching integrated into wellness benefits
- Healthy cafeteria "defaults"

> A workplace should operate like that Paris park, a place where movement happens naturally, socially, and without friction.

Design Principle #4: Government Incentives = National Nudges

Governments already subsidize medications. Why not subsidize prevention?

Effective interventions:

- Gym-membership tax credits
- Wearable-device rebates
- Insurance rewards for meeting step goals
- Funding for outdoor gyms in every city
- National campaigns: "Walk 10 Minutes After Meals"
- School programs teaching metabolic health

These incentives mimic exactly what made that Paris morning powerful: environmental momentum.

Nudging: Gentle Forces, Massive Impact

Thaler and Sunstein define a nudge as a design change that influences behaviour without restricting choice.[14] That Paris outdoor gym was a nudge. The pathways were nudges. The bike lanes were nudges.

Nudges are inexpensive but remarkably effective.

Nudge #1: Outdoor Movement Nudges

Examples Canada could adopt:

- Outdoor calisthenics zones in every major park
- "Movement Loops" with step counts posted
- Well-lit trails for year-round walking
- Public "10-minute post-meal walk" signage

Just like my family did in Paris, spontaneous movement emerges in well-designed spaces.

Nudge #2: Food Nudges

Behavioural science shows small changes create massive shifts:[15]

TABLE 4 – Effective Public-Health Nudges

Nudge	Impact	Evidence
Fruit at eye level	↑ fruit purchases 25–40%	Sunstein/ Thaler
Healthy defaults	↑ screening, ↑ healthy choices	Patel et al., NEJM
Social norm text nudges	↑ steps by 700–1,200/day	Milkman et al., PNAS
Sleep wind-down prompts	↑ sleep by 30–45 mins	Chang et al., PNAS

Restaurants and grocery stores can apply this with minimal cost:

- Place whole foods at entrances
- Promote protein-first meals
- Create “green muscle” sections emphasizing strength foods

This is choice architecture. Not forcing, just shaping.

Nudge #3: Sleep & Stress Nudges

Our environment currently works against sleep.

Screens. Light pollution. Stress.

Changes that work:

- Automatic phone wind-down modes
- “No screens one hour before sleep” workplace campaigns
- Magnesium and relaxation kits in corporate wellness programs
- Light dimming in public spaces after 9 p.m.

Better sleep reduces inflammation, improves metabolic health, and protects mental health.[16]

Nudge #4: Metabolic Health Nudges

Wearables + behavioural science = a prevention revolution:

- Post-meal walking reminders
- Protein-intake nudges
- Automatic booking of A1C and lipid screening
- Insurance incentives for improved step trends

If a Paris park can nudge a tourist family into a full workout, imagine what structured nudges could do for an entire nation.

The Paris Model as a Blueprint for Canada

The morning my family worked out in that Paris park wasn't an "exercise session." It was public health in action.

A city that:

- normalizes movement
- encourages connection
- embeds strength training
- values walkability
- integrates fitness across generations

Those principles can, and must, guide Canadian health reform.

TABLE 5 – Outdoor Gyms: International Examples

City	Outdoor Gyms	Annual Users	Outcome
Paris	1,200+	3M+	Movement normalized
Barcelona	800+	1.5M	Active aging supported
Sydney	600+	1.2M	Family participation ↑
Vancouver	120+	350k	Strong senior uptake
Toronto	~100	300k	High-growth potential

These are not luxuries. These are investments that prevent chronic disease far more effectively than medications.

Imagine a country where:

- ✓ Every neighbourhood is walkable
- ✓ Every park has an outdoor gym
- ✓ Every workplace reinforces health
- ✓ Every school teaches metabolic literacy
- ✓ Every grocery store defaults to whole foods
- ✓ Every citizen receives helpful nudges
- ✓ Every city embraces movement as culture

This isn't utopian. It's strategic. And it creates the exact conditions that made my family's Paris workout feel inevitable and joyful.

Final Thoughts

That Paris morning showed me something profound: When you build environments that support health, people naturally become healthier.

No lectures. No guilt. No massive programs. Just good design and gentle nudges.

Our job is to bring that same architecture of health to Canada. A future where health happens not because people fight for it, but because every street, workplace, school, and community supports it effortlessly.

A future where families across Canada can stumble into their own version of that Paris park...and move together like it's the most natural thing in the world.

Because it should be.

Reflection

1. What environments in your life make the healthy choice easier, and which ones make it harder?
2. If you could redesign one workplace, school, hospital, or community space to promote health, what would you change first?

Key Takeaways

- Healthy choices should be the default choices, built into our communities.
- Health is beyond an individual responsibility.
- Systems should be designed to naturally support healthier behaviors.

Chapter 7
Mental Health: The Invisible Pandemic

"Your mind is part of your health, not separate from it."

- Dr. Kwadwo Kyeremanteng

Mental health is not a luxury. It's not a niche specialty. It's not something people should have to "figure out on their own." It is foundational to human health, human functioning, and human relationships. Yet we treat it as optional, something people can access only if they can pay, wait, or reach crisis.

As an ICU physician, I've seen the consequences of this approach. I've seen young adults, parents, and seniors fall through the cracks, not because they didn't care about their health, but because support wasn't available when they needed it. And by the time they reached my unit, the damage was often irreversible.

A Story That Should Never Happen Again

He was 28 years old, bright, creative, kind, and soft-spoken. The kind of young man everyone described as "the glue" of his family. When COVID hit, his world collapsed. Work dried up. Routines disappeared. Social circles shrank. He spent months caring for his younger siblings and trying to hold himself together.

Over time, the isolation and uncertainty eroded his mental health. He wasn't sleeping. His appetite disappeared. His motivation evaporated. But like many young people, he didn't want to worry his family or friends. He blamed himself for feeling this way. He tried to get help.

He searched for a psychologist, but $180–$220 per session was out of reach.

He looked into publicly funded therapy, but the waitlist was close to a year.

He went to a walk-in counselling clinic, but they provided only short-term triage.

He wasn't in crisis, yet, so there was no immediate pathway to care.

His depression deepened. And one night, during a severe downturn, he harmed himself in a way that caused profound medical damage. When he arrived in the ICU, he was in shock, severely dehydrated, and in acute kidney failure from muscle breakdown. His heart rhythm was unstable. He survived, but he left the hospital requiring months of rehabilitation and long-term medical follow-up.

Not because he didn't try. Not because psychiatrists or clinicians failed him; they never had the chance to help. Not because he was weak. It happened because care was inaccessible until the moment everything collapsed.

His story is heartbreaking, and even more heartbreaking is how common it is. We should never accept this as normal.

Why Mental Health Must Be Universal Healthcare

We cannot continue treating mental health as secondary. Every aspect of health is shaped by mental well-being: sleep, metabolic health, recovery from illness, medication adherence, relationships, work, and overall functioning.

Here's why mental health must become a core pillar of universal healthcare:

1. Mental illness is the leading cause of disability

In Canada and globally, mental illness, especially depression and anxiety, is the number one cause of disability. Not cancer. Not heart disease. Mental illness.

It leads to:

- more lost work days
- more disability claims
- more early retirements
- more family strain
- more economic burden

For young adults, nothing drives disability more than mental illness.

2. Mental illness worsens physical health

Mental health is not separate from physical health.

Depression and anxiety worsen:

- diabetes control
- heart outcomes
- chronic pain
- medication adherence
- sleep quality
- recovery after surgery

Patients with mental illness stay longer in hospital, re-admit more often, and have worse outcomes.

3. ERs and ICUs absorb the consequences

> Emergency departments have become the de facto mental health access point.

That was never the plan, but it's reality.

We routinely see:

- suicide attempts
- intentional or accidental overdoses
- self-neglect leading to severe infection
- anxiety presenting as chest pain
- psychosis triggered by stress or substance use

By the time someone reaches the ICU, the system has already failed them.

4. The economic burden is massive

A conservative estimate places Canada's total annual cost of mental illness at $53–70 billion.

Table 1. Estimated Annual Cost of Mental Illness in Canada

(CIHI, CAMH, MHCC)

Category	Estimated Cost	Notes
Direct healthcare	$11–13B	ER visits, hospital stays, outpatient services
Lost productivity	$39–42B	Absenteeism, disability, reduced performance
Premature mortality	$6–7B	Suicide, overdose
Social services & justice	$7–8B	Housing, policing, shelters
Total	$53–70B/year	Conservative estimate

Mental health is not "too expensive to treat universally." Not treating it is what's expensive.

The Modern Mental Health Storm: Phones, Sleep, and Isolation

We are living in an environment that is hostile to mental well-being.

1. Smartphones disrupt recovery

Constant notifications keep the brain activated, preventing the parasympathetic nervous system from doing its job: rest, recovery, regulation.

2. Social media fuels comparison and loneliness

Everyone feels behind. Everyone feels inadequate. The highlight-reel effect hits young people especially hard.

3. Sleep is deteriorating

A decade ago, teenagers slept around 8–9 hours a night. Today, many barely hit 6–7. Sleep deprivation increases:

- anxiety
- depression
- impulsivity
- risk-taking
- emotional reactivity
- cravings and poor nutrition

Sleep is medicine. Without it, everything falls apart.

Metabolic Health and Mental Health: One System, Not Two

One of the most overlooked connections in medicine is the link between metabolic dysfunction and mental illness. If you want to improve mental health across a population, you must improve metabolic health.

Metabolic dysfunction increases the risk of:

- depression
- anxiety
- chronic fatigue

- cognitive slowing
- ADHD-like symptoms
- emotional instability

Conversely, exercise, sleep regulation, protein-forward nutrition, and strength training are powerful mood stabilizers. This is not just physical health, but a mental health strategy.

Prevention Must Begin in Schools

If we want generational change, we must start early.

Schools should teach:

- emotional regulation
- stress-management techniques
- sleep literacy
- physical activity as medicine
- how to recognize depressive symptoms
- how to ask for help
- the effects of processed food and screen time
- simple self-care practices
- daily movement habits

If we taught mental health skills the way we teach reading, we would prevent thousands of crises every year.

Technology as Prevention: Mindstride and Beyond

The future of mental health is early detection. Technology can detect subtle changes before people consciously realize they're struggling:

- declining sleep duration
- lower HRV
- less communication with friends
- reduced physical activity
- irregular routines
- language pattern changes
- increased late-night screen time

Platforms like Mindstride can nudge early:

- "Your sleep is trending low. Try tonight's 5-minute wind-down."
- "Let's do a short breathing exercise."
- "Your stress markers are rising. Check in with yourself."
- "Go for a walk. It will lower your cortisol."

AI will not replace therapy or clinicians, but it can provide early, continuous support between human encounters. It's the future of scalable prevention.

VIPA: How We Fix Mental Health

Real reform requires clarity, courage, and coordination. This is how we move from crisis-driven care to prevention-driven systems.

V – VALUES: The Foundation of Change

Values determine what we build. If we value:

- dignity
- equity
- early access
- prevention
- affordability
- compassion

...then mental health must be treated as core healthcare. Stating our values makes the path forward obvious: Mental health is healthcare. Mental health is universal. Mental health is prevention. These are ethical commitments, not slogans.

I – INTEGRATIVE THINKING: Creating Better Solutions

Roger Martin's integrative thinking reminds us we don't need to choose between imperfect options. We can create better ones.

Right now, mental health is full of false choices:

- ✗ Public system OR private counsellors
- ✗ Therapy OR medication
- ✗ Virtual OR in-person
- ✗ Crisis response OR prevention
- ✗ School-based care OR primary care

Integrative thinking says:

Why not both?

Why not all?

Why not a blended system that takes the best of each?

This is how we build:

- ✓ School-based screening + tech nudges + rapid follow-up
- ✓ Primary care with embedded mental health workers
- ✓ Affordable virtual care + in-person therapy when needed

✓ Metabolic interventions + counselling + medication when appropriate

✓ Public funding + employer partnerships + community supports

It's the Toronto International Film Festival model: taking the best of accessibility, excellence, and global recognition, not choosing between extremes, but integrating them.

P – PARETO & PSYCHOLOGICAL SAFETY: Pulling a Few Levers

Two critical elements:

1. The Pareto Principle (80/20)

If 80% of outcomes come from 20% of actions, then we must focus on the interventions that move the needle. The high-impact 20% includes:

- early identification
- rapid access
- affordable therapy
- exercise and strength training
- sleep regulation
- nutrition

- connection
- tech-enabled monitoring
- school-based literacy

These few levers prevent thousands of crises and ICU admissions.

2. Psychological Safety

People must feel safe saying:

"I'm struggling."

"I need help."

"I can't afford therapy."

"I'm overwhelmed."

Psychological safety must exist in:

- workplaces
- families
- schools
- sports teams
- healthcare teams

Without it, people hide their pain until crisis is the only access point. That is the system we have now, and the system we must leave behind.

A – ACTION: Turning Vision Into Reality

Values are meaningless without execution. Integration is meaningless without follow-through.

This is where change happens.

System-Level Actions

- Publicly funded or subsidized therapy
- Mental health workers in every primary care clinic
- Annual school-based mental health checks
- Expanded crisis services
- Tech platforms for early detection
- National virtual CBT programs
- Integration of mental and metabolic health

Community Actions

- Mental health literacy programs
- Employer-funded access to therapy
- Peer support networks
- Community gyms and movement programs

Individual Actions

- Daily movement
- Sleep consistency
- Strength training
- Simple nutrition
- Connection
- Early help-seeking
- Leveraging tech for insight and prevention

VIPA turns a massive, overwhelming societal challenge into something clear, structured, and actionable.

Values tell us why.

Integration tells us how.

Pareto and safety tell us where to focus.

Action makes it real.

Final Thoughts

We are living through an invisible pandemic of loneliness, depression, anxiety, burnout, and hopelessness. But this crisis is not inevitable. It is absolutely solvable.

If we embed our values into policy...

If we embrace integrative thinking...

If we focus on the highest-impact levers...

If we build psychological safety...

If we take action: real, coordinated, preventative action...

...then we will build a society where young people do not fall through the cracks, where early help is accessible, where mental health care is universal, and where stories like the one that opened this chapter become rare, not routine.

Mental health is healthcare. Mental health is prevention. And mental health is the future of a thriving, resilient population.

Reflection

1. How would our healthcare system change if mental health was treated as foundational, not optional?
2. What would earlier, easier, and more compassionate mental health support look like in your community?

Key Takeaways

- Metabolic health and mental health are inseparable.
- Mental health must become fully integrated into universal healthcare.
- Early access prevents crisis, disability, and medical complications.

Chapter 8

The Unsung Heroes of Flow: Physios, Social Workers & Discharge Planners

---

"Hospitals do not flow because of beds.
They flow because of people."

- Dr. Kwadwo Kyeremanteng

One of the most impressive things I witnessed early in my career was at Quinte Health in Belleville. On their wards, they had extra physiotherapists, social workers, and a proactive discharge-planning team.

Sometimes, they'd come to me and say, "Dr. K, Mrs. X is ready for discharge. We've already organized her home care and follow-ups. All you need to do is sign the note."

It was beautiful.

In most hospitals, that kind of efficiency feels like fiction. But at Quinte, it was normal, and it transformed care. Patients moved through the system faster, morale was higher, and everyone worked in sync. It was one of the first times I saw what true interdisciplinary collaboration could do.

I'll never forget Mr. S, a retired mechanic in his late seventies admitted with pneumonia. He'd survived the infection, but weeks in bed had left him frail, unable to walk even a few steps without support. In another setting, he might have stayed weeks longer, waiting for rehab, waiting for home care, waiting for someone to decide what to do next. But not here.

Within hours, the **physiotherapist** had him sitting up, standing, and taking his first steps. The **social worker** arranged a home safety assessment and lined up community physiotherapy. The **discharge planner** secured transportation and follow-up appointments.

Three days later, he was walking, slowly, but proudly, out of the hospital. Months afterward, I ran into him at the grocery store. He was pushing his cart, chatting about his grandkids, and told me, "Doc, those physios saved my life." He wasn't exaggerating. In modern medicine, survival is often the easy part. Regaining function, that's the battle.

The First to Be Cut, Yet the Most Valuable

Too often, the first positions cut when budgets tighten are physiotherapists, occupational therapists, and discharge planners. On paper, they're seen as "support staff." In reality, they are the capacity creators, the people who keep the system flowing.

Physiotherapists don't just help people move. They restore independence, confidence, and dignity. In critical care, I've seen countless patients who survived the illness but never recovered the ability to stand or walk. And once function is lost, everything spirals: complications increase, readmissions rise, and long-term care placements follow. Physios fight that decline every single day. They are the frontline defense against frailty, the hidden epidemic that quietly drains our healthcare system.

And our social workers and discharge planners? They carry an emotional weight few appreciate. They navigate family tensions, organize home care, secure medical equipment, and coordinate dozens of small details that determine whether a patient can safely go home. Their compassion and logistics skills often spell the difference between a smooth transition and a revolving hospital door.

When I think of system heroes, I don't picture the latest surgical robot or medication. I picture these teams working quietly, solving problems, keeping humanity in the system.

Function Is Medicine

One of the strongest predictors of survival after illness isn't the medication used. It's mobility, the ability to get out of bed, to walk, to maintain strength. In other words, function is medicine. And function doesn't come from a pill. It comes from movement, from confidence, from early rehabilitation.

Every day a patient stays in bed, they lose strength. For older adults, one extra day immobile can mean the loss of independence. By prioritizing mobility from day one, physiotherapists literally change outcomes. A system that values function values life.

How Proactive Discharge Changes Everything

At Quinte, the discharge-planning team didn't wait for instructions; they anticipated needs. They rounded daily, identified barriers early, and coordinated community services before discharge was even discussed.

Because of that approach:

- Length of stay dropped
- Weekend discharges increased
- Families felt informed instead of blindsided
- Staff felt less burned out and more supported

It was elegant, simple, and profoundly effective. They weren't reacting. They were leading.

A Future Built on Flow

If we want to improve efficiency in healthcare, we must invest in flow: the movement of patients through the system, safely and seamlessly. Imagine every hospital having a dedicated flow team: physiotherapists, occupational therapists, social workers, and discharge specialists who coordinate transitions in real time.

Now imagine adding AI-assisted dashboards that predict who's trending toward readiness for discharge, who's at risk of deterioration, and where bottlenecks are forming. A centralized command center could oversee these patterns across multiple sites, ensuring that beds, equipment, and staff are used where they're needed most.

That's not science fiction. It's what happens when we blend human compassion with data-driven insight.

The Economics of Common Sense

Every unnecessary hospital day costs the system hundreds, sometimes thousands, of dollars. Multiply that across thousands of patients, and you're looking at millions in avoidable costs. Adding one physiotherapist or discharge planner can pay for itself many times over in reduced length of stay, improved outcomes, and fewer readmissions.

Cutting these roles may make a quarterly report look tidy, but it cripples flow and costs far more in the long run.

> If we truly want sustainable healthcare, we must redefine what "essential" means.

It's not just doctors, nurses, and diagnostics. It's the people who help patients get home safely and stay home. We need to stop treating these professions as extras and start recognizing them as the backbone of efficiency, humanity, and patient experience.

A Vision for Tomorrow

Picture a health system where every admission includes a discharge plan from day one. Physiotherapists track mobility goals, social workers engage families early, and discharge planners coordinate everything from follow-up appointments to equipment delivery.

Overlay this with AI support: real-time monitoring of patient readiness, community capacity, and flow patterns. Patients move smoothly through care. Families feel supported. Clinicians get to focus on healing instead of chasing paperwork. That's not just efficient healthcare, but compassionate design.

Final Thoughts

When I think back to my time in Belleville, I realize I was witnessing the future. A system where collaboration, anticipation, and empathy drive efficiency. If we want to fix healthcare, we don't need more bureaucracy or bigger hospitals. We need to reinvest in people who restore function and create flow.

Because at the end of the day, better flow means better care, and better care means better lives.

Reflection

1. Who are the overlooked people in your organization who quietly keep patients moving, healing, and safe?
2. What would happen if we invested more intentionally in the teams that prevent bottlenecks instead of only reacting to them?

Key Takeaways

- Functional recovery is just as important as survival.
- Interdisciplinary teamwork improves healthcare flow.
- Coordinated discharge planning reduces readmissions.

Part III

Driving Forward Momentum

Chapter 9
One EMR: Connecting the Dots

"If you can't share information, you can't share care."

- Dr. Kwadwo Kyeremanteng

The fact that we still don't have a single, unified electronic medical record (EMR) across a province is, frankly, baffling. In an age where I can send money instantly to someone on the other side of the world, we still struggle to send a patient's CT scan across town.

Every day in the ICU, I see the cost of this fragmentation, financial, operational, and human. Patients arrive from other hospitals, long-term care facilities, or clinics, and too often, we're left with incomplete information. Their medications, allergies, lab results, or prior imaging aren't accessible. We start from scratch, sometimes literally repeating expensive tests that were done just days earlier.

These inefficiencies are more than an inconvenience; they represent systemic waste and clinical risk. Every redundant CT scan, lab draw, or consultation costs the system thousands of dollars and drains precious time. But beyond the dollars, it can delay care, and sometimes, that delay has devastating consequences.

When Communication Breaks Down

A middle-aged man came to our ICU from a regional hospital with what looked like a severe infection. He had been started on broad-spectrum antibiotics, but we didn't have access to his cultures, imaging, or lab trends. We didn't even know whether his infection had already been imaged or if his antibiotics had been changed recently.

Because of that lack of information, we ordered a repeat CT scan. The result confirmed what his original imaging, done just 36 hours earlier, had already shown. We lost time, resources, and momentum. Thankfully, he recovered, but it was a reminder that these gaps in communication aren't abstract. They affect real people, real outcomes.

Now multiply that by the hundreds of thousands of patient transfers, referrals, and consultations happening daily across a province, and you start to see the scale of the problem.

A Patchwork System

Healthcare in most provinces is a patchwork of platforms, different hospitals, clinics, and regions using different EMRs that rarely "talk" to each other. Even within one city, you can have half a dozen systems operating independently.

That means physicians often rely on phone calls, faxes, or patients' memories to piece together a medical history. It's inefficient, archaic, and risky. In 2025, this is simply unacceptable.

> A healthcare system that can't communicate within itself is like a body that's lost its nervous system.

The left hand doesn't know what the right hand is doing.

The Case for One Record

Yes, implementing a single provincial EMR is expensive. The initial cost can be measured in hundreds of millions, sometimes billions. But that's only one side of the equation. The cost of not doing it, in duplication, errors, burnout, and poor outcomes, is far greater.

A unified EMR is not a luxury; it's infrastructure. The same way we invest in roads, bridges, and broadband internet, we must invest in the digital infrastructure that connects our healthcare system. When we do, here's what's possible:

- ✓ **Seamless communication** across all levels of care, from primary care to hospitals, rehab centers, and home care.
- ✓ **Reduced duplication** of imaging, labs, and diagnostics, saving the system millions annually.
- ✓ **Better patient safety** through shared medication lists and allergy records.
- ✓ **Empowered patients** who can access their own data, book appointments, and track results.
- ✓ **Richer research data** to drive innovation, identify trends, and create predictive models that personalize care.

In other words, it's not just about saving time, but saving lives.

Innovation Through Integration

A single EMR does more than improve logistics. It unlocks the future of medicine. Imagine being able to analyze patterns across millions of anonymized patient records to predict who's at risk for heart failure, diabetes, or cancer before symptoms even begin. Imagine AI models that alert your primary care team when subtle changes in your lab work suggest metabolic decline, or when someone's blood pressure trends upward across visits.

With one connected system, we can move from reactive care to proactive care, from treatment to prevention. That's the essence of healthcare reform. And it's not hypothetical. Alberta is already moving in this direction with its Connect Care system. Quebec is investing heavily in a unified platform, and several other provinces have begun pilot projects. Ontario has taken steps with regional digital health networks, but we need to accelerate.

The technology exists. The leadership will determine whether we seize this opportunity or remain stuck in fragmentation.

The Patient Experience

Let's not forget the patient.

For patients, navigating the healthcare system can feel like wandering through a maze with no map. They see their family doctor, go for tests at one hospital, see a specialist at another, and end up in the emergency department days later. At every step, they're asked the same questions: *What medications are you taking? When was your last test? Who's your doctor?*

A unified EMR would eliminate that burden. Patients could log in to one portal, see their records, and even share them with new providers. This transparency fosters trust and engagement. When people understand and can access their own data, they become partners in their care, not just passengers.

From Data to Wisdom

Healthcare generates massive amounts of data, but without integration, that data sits in silos, underutilized and often invisible. A single EMR would allow us to turn data into wisdom: to learn what's working, identify risks earlier, and measure the impact of interventions. It would transform quality improvement, public health planning, and even clinical education.

And for research, the implications are enormous. We could finally conduct large-scale, real-time studies without waiting years for data linkage. We could test what works in real-world settings, accelerating discovery and innovation. This is the kind of infrastructure that doesn't just modernize healthcare, but propels it.

Ultimately, a single EMR is about connection: connecting people, teams, and systems. It's about ensuring that wherever a patient goes within a province, their story follows them. Healthcare is complex, but communication doesn't have to be. We've done this before. We've connected banking, transportation, and communication networks across entire countries. We can connect healthcare too. It simply requires the will.

The Cost of Inaction

Every year we delay, we pay the price in inefficiency, frustration, and worse outcomes. We waste money on duplicate tests, we lose opportunities for early detection, and we burn out healthcare workers who spend hours chasing information that should be a click away.

We can't afford to keep patching holes in a fragmented system. It's time to build something unified, smart, and enduring.

Final Thoughts

If we're serious about improving healthcare delivery, this is one of the most impactful steps we can take. A single provincial EMR will not solve all our problems, but it will make nearly every other solution easier. It's the foundation on which better communication, continuity, and innovation can be built.

When every provider can see the same information, every patient gets better care. When every patient can access their data, they gain agency. And when the system learns from its collective data, healthcare finally evolves. This isn't just a digital upgrade. It's a paradigm shift.

One province. One record. One patient story.

That's how we connect the dots, and that's how we build a system worthy of the people it serves.

Reflection

1. Where does fragmented information currently create harm, delay, duplication, or frustration in patient care?
2. What would become possible if every clinician caring for a patient could see the same essential information at the right time?

Key Takeaways

- The standard should be one patient, one record.
- Fragmented medical records create inefficiency, duplication, and safety risks.
- Unified digital infrastructure is necessary for future healthcare reform.

Chapter 10
Public-Private Partnerships: A Pragmatic Path to Faster Care, Better Outcomes, and a Stronger Healthcare System

---

"If we truly believe in universal healthcare, then we must also believe in doing whatever works."

- Dr. Kwadwo Kyeremanteng

He was in his late seventies, a retired teacher with the kind of energy most twenty-year-olds would envy. For decades, his routine was sacred: three rounds of golf a week, long walks with his wife, and a firm refusal to "grow old quietly." He was one of those people who believed movement was medicine, and to be fair, he was right.

Then his hip started to go. At first, it was a nuisance. A stiffness getting out of the car. A twinge halfway through his backswing. Then a limp. Then days when the pain kicked so hard he could barely walk his dog, let alone complete a round of golf. His family doctor referred him for a hip replacement.

And then... he waited. Six months. Then nine. Then twelve.

By the time his surgery date arrived, he was nowhere near the man he had been. His muscle had melted away. His gait had become unstable. His world had shrunk to the few steps he could manage inside his home. The active, proud, independent man who once mentored students and young teachers now needed help tying his shoes.

And here's the painful truth: His decline was preventable. Not the hip deterioration. That happens. But the year he spent deteriorating on a waitlist. That was a system failure. What makes it even harder to accept is that there were surgical centers, safe, efficient, publicly funded, that could have done his hip months earlier, at a lower cost, with better flow and outcomes, but the system never routed him there.

This is the cost of a system that confuses ideology with healthcare delivery. This is why we must talk openly about public-private partnerships.

The Efficiency Gap: What Specialized Centres Can Do That Hospitals Can't

Let's be very clear from the start: this is not about privatizing healthcare. It is not about two-tier care. It is not about American-style anything. This is about leveraging publicly funded procedures delivered in high-efficiency centers that can dramatically increase capacity, shorten wait lists, and improve outcomes, without charging patients out of pocket.

We already do this. We've just been too timid about scaling it.

A typical Canadian academic hospital performs around 3–4 joint replacements per OR per day.

A specialized orthopedic surgical center routinely performs 6–8 safely and consistently (CIHI Wait Times Report, 2023).

Why the difference?

Because while hospitals deal with traumas, emergencies, unstable medical patients, staffing shortages, and bed constraints, specialized centers are designed for predictable, lower-complexity procedures that run like a Formula 1 pit crew. Everyone knows their role. Turnover is fast. Equipment is standardized. Patients flow.

Shouldice Hospital, Canada's iconic hernia center, is the perfect example. They've been repairing hernias for over half a century with:

- minimal complications
- short stays
- high patient satisfaction
- and exceptional throughput

All while billing the public system (Shouldice Annual Report, 2023). This is what efficiency looks like when done well. And it isn't theoretical. It's happening right now, in Canada, within medicare.

The False Dichotomy Holding Us Back

For too long, healthcare debates in Canada have been framed as a binary choice: public good vs. private involvement. But that is a false dichotomy.

Every modern healthcare system, U.K., France, Australia, Sweden, uses a mix of public and private delivery while maintaining universal access (OECD Health at a Glance, 2022). The patient doesn't care who owns the brick and mortar.

The patient cares about:

- timely care
- safe outcomes
- competent professionals
- and getting their life back

The reality is simple:

Public funding + private or specialized delivery = faster, safer, more efficient care.

This is not a threat to medicare. It is a lifeline for it.

Data Tables (Conservative Estimates)

(CIHI, OECD, Shouldice Hospital, Alberta Surgical Initiative, Kensington Eye Institute; compiled 2022–2024)

Table 1. Academic Hospitals vs. Specialized Surgical Centres

Metric	Academic Hospital (Typical)	Specialized Centre	Notes
Hip/Knee Replacements per OR per Day	3–4	6–8	Conservative estimate
Cataract Surgeries per Day	10–14	18–24	High efficiency

Minor Surgeries per Day	5-7	12-20	Local anesthesia advantage
Turnover Time	25-45 min	8-15 min	Dedicated staff
Cost per Joint Replacement	$10k-$12.5k	$8k-$10k	Lower overhead
Cost per Cataract	$1.2k-$1.5k	$750-$1k	Predictable workflow
Cancellation Rate	5-15%	<2%	Hospitals face emergencies
Same-Day Discharge	25-50%	60-90%	Enhanced recovery pathways

Table 2. Orthopedic Efficiency

Metric	Academic Hospital	Specialized Centre
Hip Replacements per Day	2-3	4-5
Knee Replacements per Day	2-3	4-6
Turnover Time	30-45 min	10-20 min
Readmission Rate	4-7%	3-5%
Median Wait Time	6-16 months	3-8 months

Table 3. Ophthalmology Efficiency

Metric	Academic Hospital	Specialized Eye Centre
Cataracts per OR per Day	10-14	18-24

Turnover Time	15-25 min	6-10 min
Complication Rate	1-1.5%	0.6-1%
Wait Time	4-12 months	2-5 months

Table 4. Minor Surgery Efficiency

Procedure	Academic Throughput	Specialized Centre
Carpal Tunnel	4-6 per day	8-12 per day
Hernia Repair	3-5 per day	6-10 per day
Skin Lesions	15-25 per day	25-40 per day
Port Insertions	4-6 per day	6-12 per day
Cancellation Rate	5-10%	1-3%

What Exactly Is "Minor Surgery"?

Minor surgery refers to low-risk, high-volume procedures that:

- do not require overnight hospitalization
- have predictable case durations
- have low complication rates
- are often performed with local anesthetic or light sedation
- are extremely well suited to high-efficiency centers

Examples include:

- carpal tunnel release
- trigger finger release
- ganglion cyst excision
- simple hernia repairs
- skin cancers and lesion removals
- port insertions for oncology
- varicose vein procedures
- tonsillectomies and adenoidectomies (in select centers)

These procedures should never be competing with trauma cases, ICU admissions, or emergencies for OR time. Yet that is exactly what happens in large academic hospitals. And that is why minor surgeries are among the most backlogged in Canada (CIHI Priority Procedures Report, 2023).

Public–Private Partnerships Strengthen Hospitals, Not Replace Them

Contrary to popular fear, shifting appropriate surgeries to specialized centers does not weaken hospitals. It liberates them.

1. Hospitals gain capacity for complex cases

When routine cases move off-site, hospitals can focus on trauma, ICU patients, cancer surgeries, and high-acuity care.

2. Emergency pressures decrease

Fewer elective cases means fewer cancellations and more predictable OR schedules.

3. Training environments improve

Residents and fellows get exposure to complex cases without competing with low-acuity procedures.

4. Costs decrease

High-volume, predictable procedures are cheaper to run in dedicated centers.

5. Patient flow accelerates

Waitlists drop. Quality improves. Everybody wins. This is not theoretical. Alberta, Quebec, B.C., and Nova Scotia have already demonstrated it (Alberta Surgical Initiative, 2023; Quebec IPSC Data, 2022).

What Other Countries Already Do (and We Can Learn From)

We are not the first country to face surgical backlog challenges.

United Kingdom

The U.K. uses Independent Sector Treatment Centres (ISTCs) to deliver publicly funded surgeries when NHS capacity is strained. They've reduced wait times while maintaining universal access (NHS England, 2022).

Australia

Australia blends public funding with private surgical delivery for elective procedures. Universal coverage remains intact, and wait times have consistently been lower than Canada's (Australian Institute of Health and Welfare, 2022).

Sweden & Netherlands

Both countries use privately owned but publicly funded surgical centers for cataracts, orthopedics, and minor surgery, dramatically increasing throughput and shortening waits.

We are behind not because we lack the talent or the resources, but because we lack the willingness to innovate.

A VIPA Framework for Modernizing Surgical Capacity

This is where the VIPA framework comes in: Values, Integrative Thinking, Pareto, Action.

Values

The value that defines universal healthcare is timely access, not maintaining outdated structures. If a patient waits a year for a surgery that could be delivered safely in a month, that is not equity.

That is harm.

Integrative Thinking

We don't have to choose between public and private. We choose both, strategically. We create a Canadian model that selects the best of each world:

- the equity and universality of public funding
- the efficiency and focus of specialized centers

- the oversight and accountability of health ministries
- the nimbleness and innovation of non-hospital providers

This is integrative thinking in action.

Pareto Principle (80/20)

If just 20–30% of minor, orthopedic, and ophthalmologic surgeries were shifted to specialized centers, we could reduce waitlists by 40–60% nationally (CIHI projections, 2023). One targeted intervention could transform the system.

Action

We cannot debate this into the ground. We need pilots, partnerships, outcome measurement. We need courage. And we need it now.

The Real Cost of Doing Nothing

If we continue with the status quo:

- more patients will suffer functional decline
- more older adults will lose independence
- more people will fall into frailty

- more caregivers will burn out
- more preventable complications will arise
- more money will be wasted on hospital inefficiencies

A hip that waits 12 months costs more than a hip done at three months, not just financially, but in human suffering. As an ICU physician, I see what happens when people fall into frailty. They stay in hospital longer, require more rehab, and lose independence. Their quality of life diminishes. Prevention is always cheaper than rescue.

Let's return to our golfer.

Imagine a system where:

- his surgery is routed to a high-volume orthopedic center
- he receives care within weeks
- he maintains function
- he keeps golfing
- he stays strong, independent, and engaged in life

That should be the norm in Canada, not the exception. Public-private partnerships are not about profit or ideology. They are about preserving function, dignity, and quality of life. They are about delivering on the true promise of universal healthcare.

Final Thoughts

Canada's healthcare system is full of passionate people, physicians, nurses, administrators, policymakers, who want to do the right thing. But we are often working within structures that were designed decades ago, for a population and healthcare burden that no longer exists.

We cannot rely on a single delivery model to solve modern challenges.

We need boldness. We need innovation.

We need humility to adopt what works, wherever it lives.

We need courage to move past ideology and into action.

Public-private partnerships are not a betrayal of Canadian values. They are an expression of them. Universal healthcare is not about maintaining a specific delivery model, but about ensuring that every Canadian receives timely, safe, high-quality care.

And if specialized centers can deliver that ,with public dollars, within a universal framework, then it is not just acceptable. It is essential. This is the path to shorter waitlists. This is the path to improved outcomes. This is the path to keeping people strong, functional, and independent. This is the path to a healthier Canada. And it starts with the courage to say:

We will do whatever works.

Reflection

1. Where could a responsible public-private partnership improve access while still protecting fairness and universal care?
2. What safeguards would need to be in place for innovation to strengthen the public system rather than undermine it?

Key Takeaways

- Public-private partnerships can strengthen, not replace, universal healthcare.
- Hospitals should focus on high-acuity care while lower-risk procedures move to streamlined centers.
- High-efficiency centers reduce wait times, costs, and cancellations.

Chapter 11

Innovation: The Engine of a Healthcare System Ready for the Future

---

"Healthcare doesn't just need more resources. It needs more ideas, more connection, and more courage."

- Dr. Kwadwo Kyeremanteng

Healthcare is full of dedicated people, world-class researchers, and incredible science. But for all our talent, we still struggle to keep pace with what patients need. Not because we lack intelligence or heart, but because we lack structures that reward innovation.

We try to solve tomorrow's problems with yesterday's tools. It's why emergency departments are overflowing, why clinicians burn out, why chronic disease keeps rising, and why technologies that could transform care never make it past pilot projects.

To change this, every region, every hospital, and every health network must have an innovation hub, a physical and cultural home where frontline clinicians, scientists, engineers, entrepreneurs, technology builders, and investors come together to solve real problems.

Not someday.

Not in 10 years.

Now.

This is the belief that led us to create LionHeart Innovation.

Why Innovation Hubs Matter

Innovation is often mistaken for research. Research is essential, but it is slow. Painfully slow. A discovery in a lab can take 10–17 years to reach clinical practice.

Meanwhile:

- patients wait
- clinicians burn out
- costs rise
- inefficiencies multiply
- chronic disease accelerates

Innovation hubs bridge the gap between discovery and deployment.

They allow us to:

- pilot solutions quickly
- test ideas in real care environments
- connect researchers with builders
- match clinicians' needs with tech capability
- support companies through regulatory and commercialization barriers

Instead of discussing the same problems for years, innovation hubs help us fix them in months. They turn frustration into action.

Clinicians Know the Problems but Need Partners to Solve Them

If you want to know where the system is failing, ask clinicians. We know the pain points because we live them:

- A patient waits 12–18 hours for a bed.
- A CT scan is repeated because we can't access previous imaging.
- A frail senior is discharged but has no home supports, leading to re-admission.

- A physician spends two hours documenting for every hour of care.
- A simple blood test requires weeks of back-and-forth for a patient with mobility issues.

Clinicians see the inefficiencies. We feel the bottlenecks. We experience the consequences. But clinicians cannot fix these problems alone.

We need engineers who can build.

Researchers who can validate.

Entrepreneurs who can iterate.

Policymakers who can enable.

Investors who can fuel growth.

Innovation hubs bring these groups together, often for the first time. This collaboration creates a multiplier effect: ideas move faster, testing is quicker, adoption improves, and impact becomes real.

The Lionheart Story: Why We Stopped Waiting and Started Building

LionHeart Innovation was not born from a business plan. It was born from frustration, and hope.

The Spark

It began with conversations among clinicians who were tired of seeing the same problems year after year, including inefficiencies, communication gaps, preventable hospitalizations, and promising startups unable to access clinical settings. Everyone had ideas, but no one had a place to test them.

No infrastructure.

No roadmap.

No pathway to execution.

In one conversation, after yet another example of avoidable inefficiency, someone said, “Why are we waiting for someone else to fix this?” The silence that followed was the answer.

Building LionHeart

LionHeart Innovation became the place that didn’t exist but desperately needed to.

A place where:

- ICU physicians sit beside AI engineers
- nurses teach founders what care really looks like
- residents and students explore ideas safely
- researchers help validate early prototypes

- venture capitalists learn directly from frontline teams
- entrepreneurs rapidly pilot and iterate solutions

LionHeart is a living laboratory, not a boardroom. It's where ideas get tested, not buried. Where failure is part of the process, not the end of it. Where clinicians reclaim ownership of innovation.

Why "LionHeart"?

Because healthcare requires courage.

Courage to challenge norms.

Courage to push for better.

Courage to innovate when the system feels stuck.

LionHeart is not just a hub. It is a mindset: Be brave enough to build the future instead of waiting for it.

eSensorum: Revolutionizing Prevention with Non-Invasive Bloodwork Patches

A powerful example of the type of innovation hubs must support is eSensorum, a Canadian company building non-invasive patches that collect and analyze blood biomarkers without traditional phlebotomy.

At the time of writing, eSensorum is seeking clinical partners, research collaborators, and investment, exactly the kind of early-stage support that innovation hubs are designed to provide.

Why Metabolic Syndrome Is the Perfect First Target

Metabolic syndrome is the silent giant driving healthcare costs and chronic disease:

- insulin resistance
- pre-diabetes and diabetes
- dyslipidemia
- hypertension
- abdominal obesity
- fatty liver
- chronic inflammation

It is upstream of:

- heart disease
- stroke
- kidney failure
- dementia
- severe infections

- poor surgical outcomes
- prolonged ICU stays

The *Prevention Over Prescription* philosophy is built on reversing this trend, but to reverse something, you must measure it. Today, most people get metabolic labs once a year, if that. By the time abnormalities appear, the damage is already done.

eSensorum Changes Everything

Imagine a world where:

- A1C trends every month, not yearly
- insulin resistance is detected years before diabetes
- lipid profiles change in real time as lifestyle improves
- inflammatory markers reveal early metabolic stress
- liver enzymes show fatty liver progression or reversal
- patients don't need to travel for bloodwork
- clinicians receive data early, not after complications

eSensorum's non-invasive patches make bloodwork effortless, continuous, actionable, and at-home. This is the holy grail of preventative care.

Why eSensorum Fits Perfectly Into an Innovation Hub

To succeed, eSensorum needs:

- a clinical site to test accuracy
- researchers to validate biomarkers
- primary care and metabolic health leaders
- integration with EMRs and digital pathways
- regulatory guidance
- commercialization support
- funding to scale

Innovation hubs make this possible by:

- accelerating pilot studies
- connecting startups to clinicians
- helping navigate Health Canada approvals
- coordinating real-world evidence
- securing investment and procurement pathways

Without a hub, companies like eSensorum face years of delay and likely leave Canada. With a hub, they can transform metabolic health here at home and globally.

The Canadian Challenge: Why Our Companies Keep Leaving

Canada is excellent at creating ideas. We are excellent at publishing research. We are excellent at training scientists and clinicians.But we struggle to commercialize. We lose our best companies because:

- procurement is slow
- regulatory pathways are unclear
- capital is limited
- provinces are fragmented
- risk tolerance is low
- pilot projects never scale
- there is no national innovation mandate

Examples of Lost Opportunities

GLP-1 drugs (Ozempic, Wegovy)

The foundational science behind these life-changing medications came from Canadian scientist Dr. Daniel Drucker, yet the commercial and economic benefits went elsewhere.

mRNA vaccine technology

Canada contributed significant early research, but lacked the ecosystem to commercialize or manufacture at scale.

Tesla origins

Canadian engineers and researchers influenced early battery and EV design, but the manufacturing and innovation ecosystem grew outside Canada.

We cannot continue exporting our potential. We must build the ecosystem that allows companies to grow here. Innovation hubs are the key.

Commercialization: The Missing Middle in Canadian Healthcare

Innovation is about execution over merely ideas. And execution requires commercialization support, which Canadian healthcare has historically lacked. Innovation hubs must help companies navigate:

- IP strategy
- regulatory pathways
- reimbursement models
- procurement processes
- real-world-evidence trials

- market access
- fundraising
- integration into clinical workflows
- national and international scale

Without commercialization infrastructure, we will always be a country of pilots, not progress.

The Timing Has Never Been Better: AI Supercharges Everything

We are entering the most exciting moment in healthcare innovation in a century.

Artificial intelligence is transforming care:

- AI scribes cutting documentation time by 70%
- predictive analytics identifying deterioration early
- algorithms optimizing OR time and bed flow
- home-hospital supported by AI-driven monitoring
- Osler AI transforming medical education
- AI nudges for vaccinations and cancer screening
- natural-language tools improving patient communication

AI is not coming; it is already here. But AI alone is not enough.

- test AI safely
- study performance
- evaluate risks
- integrate workflows
- build guardrails
- create scalable models
- ensure equity and ethical deployment

AI gives us the tools. Innovation hubs give us the runway.

The Future Belongs to the Builders

Healthcare has no shortage of problems. But it also has no shortage of talent, creativity, compassion, and ambition. What we lack is coordination, speed, and environments where ideas become reality.

Innovation hubs solve this. They are not optional. They are essential infrastructure for modern healthcare, as important as MRI machines, ICUs, or surgical suites. They turn pain points into projects, projects into pilots, pilots into solutions, and solutions into scale.

LionHeart Innovation exists because we believe clinicians must help build the future, not wait for someone else to do it. And if we build the right systems, the next eSensorum, the next Osler, the next transformative health technology will grow here, scale here, employ here, and change lives here.

This is what the future requires.

Final Thoughts

Healthcare innovation is not about apps, gadgets, or buzzwords. It is about building a system worthy of the people it serves. A system that is proactive, data-driven, connected, humane, preventative, and scalable.

Innovation hubs are how we get there. It's time to be bold. It's time to challenge the status quo. It's time to build together. Because the future of healthcare will not be built by those who complain the loudest, but by those who build the bravest.

Reflection

1. What promising healthcare ideas are currently stuck because our system does not know how to test, fund, or scale them?
2. How can we create environments where frontline clinicians, patients, researchers, and entrepreneurs solve problems together?

Key Takeaways

- Innovation hubs connect clinicians, engineers, researchers, and entrepreneurs.
- Experimentation and testing are imperative to build solutions.
- The future of healthcare depends on environments that encourage rapid implementation.

Chapter 12

AI, Flow, and the Future of Healthcare

"The future of healthcare will not be rescued by comfort. It will be built by courage."

- Dr. Kwadwo Kyeremanteng

We are standing at one of the most exciting intersections in healthcare history, where technology is finally catching up with our intentions to care better. The convergence of artificial intelligence (AI), digital health tools, and human compassion has the potential to transform a strained, reactive system into one that is proactive, predictive, and deeply personal.

For years, we have chased efficiency through paperwork and process redesigns, yet the real opportunity has arrived through intelligence and automation. AI is not just another technology trend; it is the connective tissue that can restore *flow*, between people, data, and systems, and return healthcare to its fundamental purpose: preventing suffering before it starts.

A New Era of Possibility

Across Canada and around the world, clinicians are exhausted by a system that rewards volume over value. Patients wait in hallways, nurses are stretched to the limit, and every new administrative burden pulls providers further from the bedside. Yet behind this pressure lies a profound opportunity.

AI and advanced analytics can finally help us move upstream, identifying risk earlier, preventing deterioration, and delivering care where and when it is needed most. When we integrate these technologies with compassionate leadership, we create a healthcare system that listens, learns, and adapts in real time.

Hospitals like The Ottawa Hospital are already using predictive dashboards to anticipate surges in admissions. Ontario Health's digital command centers are mapping regional capacity in real time. Internationally, Kaiser Permanente has used machine learning to reduce sepsis mortality by 25 percent, while the U.K.'s NHS is piloting AI triage tools that shorten emergency wait times. These examples are not futuristic, but the opening notes of a new era.

When Data Becomes Compassion

Several years ago, a middle-aged man came into an emergency department after his smartwatch detected an irregular heartbeat. The device was never intended to diagnose disease; it simply nudged him that something was wrong. That alert led to an ECG, which confirmed atrial fibrillation. A simple medication adjustment prevented what could have been a devastating stroke.

In another case, a woman took a photo of a mole on her arm. An AI-powered dermatology app flagged it as suspicious, prompting a biopsy that confirmed melanoma, caught early enough for curative surgery.

Stories like these show how consumer technology is transforming prevention. Wearables measure heart rate variability, recovery, and sleep quality, nudging users to move, breathe, or rest. The gentle buzz on a wrist or notification on a phone has become a micro-dose of accountability.

This quiet feedback loop builds awareness and creates a bridge between data and behavior. Health is no longer hidden in lab results or specialist offices; it is woven into daily life. And as these tools evolve, they will not just count steps. They will predict stress, inflammation, and early signs of disease.

Personalized Health: From Generic Advice to Precision Coaching

For decades, health advice has been one-size-fits-all: eat better, move more, stress less. But every person's biology, environment, and motivation are different. AI-driven personalization is closing that gap.

Today, algorithms can integrate genetics, continuous glucose monitoring, and microbiome data to create individualized nutrition plans. Apps already adjust workouts based on recovery scores and hormone cycles. A 2024 Mayo Clinic pilot found that adaptive meal-planning software improved glycemic control by 18 percent compared to standard counselling.

Gyata Nutrition and similar platforms are building this bridge between evidence and experience, pairing high-quality nutrition products with personalized digital guidance. The long-term potential is enormous: scalable prevention that respects individuality while maintaining scientific rigor.

Personalization will not replace the clinician; it will empower them. When patients arrive already tracking progress and understanding their metrics, the clinical conversation shifts from information gathering to problem solving.

Diagnosing Earlier, Treating Smarter

AI is redefining diagnostic accuracy. In radiology, algorithms trained on millions of images now match or exceed human performance in detecting early breast cancer. In pathology, digital slides analyzed by AI can highlight microscopic abnormalities invisible to the naked eye. In cardiology, machine learning models interpret ECGs to detect heart failure days before symptoms appear.

A 2023 NHS study found that AI-assisted mammography reduced false negatives by 13 percent, enabling earlier treatment for hundreds of women. Similar systems are emerging in CT interpretation, retinal scanning for diabetic disease, and voice analytics for neurological disorders.

The benefit is not merely efficiency, but equity. Rural and under-resourced regions that lack specialists can access diagnostic excellence through cloud-based AI platforms. Patients who once waited months for interpretation can receive results within hours. The technology is democratizing expertise and narrowing the gap between urban and rural health outcomes.

AI's predictive capabilities are also reshaping prevention itself. Imagine your phone or wearable not only tracking your sleep or heart rate, but also reminding you when you're due for a colonoscopy, Pap test, or flu shot based on your age, risk factors, and even local disease patterns.

This isn't far off. Some health systems are already piloting AI-driven population health tools that send personalized vaccine reminders or automatically schedule cancer screenings when new data indicates increased risk. Instead of relying on chance or memory, technology will quietly keep us on track, catching illness before it ever appears.

For a system like Canada's, where screening rates often fall short of national targets, such automation could close long-standing equity gaps. An algorithm that notices you haven't had a mammogram in four years and arranges it proactively is more than convenient. It's lifesaving prevention at scale.

Mental Health in the Digital Age

Few areas reveal the need for innovation more clearly than mental health. Wait times for therapy in Canada can exceed six months; for many, that's too late. Digital platforms such as Mindstride are stepping into this space, offering real-time nudges to journal, move, or breathe when users show signs of declining mood.

These systems analyze behavioral data (sleep, physical activity, even typing cadence) to detect early warning signs. They don't replace therapists; they extend their reach. In a recent pilot across several Canadian workplaces, Mindstride reduced reported anxiety scores by 22 percent after eight weeks. The result is a hybrid model of care that empowers the individual while keeping professionals in the loop. For clinicians, it's an upstream tool; for patients, it's a lifeline. This is what equitable access looks like when technology serves compassion.

Predicting Crisis Before It Happens

Inside hospitals, AI is becoming a silent guardian. Through waveform analysis and continuous vital sign monitoring, it can detect subtle physiological changes that precede deterioration.

Dr. Andrew Seely's company in Ottawa has pioneered technology that analyzes heart-rate variability to predict which patients are about to decline. These early-warning systems allow teams to intervene before an ICU transfer becomes necessary. The cost savings are immense. Avoiding a single ICU admission can save $50,000, and each day outside the unit spares patients from the physical and psychological toll of critical illness.

At The Ottawa Hospital, our Virtual Critical Care program builds on this model. Smaller regional hospitals can connect instantly with ICU specialists via telemedicine, using AI-assisted monitoring to identify at-risk patients. The result is fewer emergency transfers, faster treatment, and patients who remain close to home.

This is the power of technology: democratizing expertise while restoring local autonomy.

Hospital at Home: Care Without Walls

One of the most promising evolutions in modern care is the Hospital-at-Home model. Patients recovering from heart failure, pneumonia, or post-surgical conditions can now receive continuous remote monitoring and daily clinician check-ins from their own homes.

Studies from the U.S. Veterans Health Administration show 25–30 percent cost reductions and equivalent or better clinical outcomes. Ontario's initial hospital-at-home pilots are showing similar promise. AI plays a central role, interpreting streams of biometric data, flagging changes, and coordinating logistics. When oxygen saturation dips or blood pressure trends upward, the system alerts the care team instantly.

These programs turn homes into micro-wards supported by digital infrastructure, allowing patients to heal in the most comfortable environment possible. The implications are vast: reduced hospital congestion, fewer infections, shorter lengths of stay, and a patient experience grounded in dignity.

Smarter Systems, Smoother Flow

Healthcare's greatest challenge is not always medicine, but movement. Beds, referrals, and discharges form a complex ecosystem that too often collapses under its own weight.

AI can restore that flow. Predictive analytics can identify which patients are ready for discharge, which require observation, and which should be prioritized for specialist review. Ontario Health's regional dashboards are already using real-time data to balance load across hospitals, preventing overcrowding in one site while others have capacity.

In the U.S., Kaiser Permanente's AI-driven scheduling platform reduced average emergency-department length of stay by 17 percent. The NHS uses similar forecasting to predict hospital occupancy days in advance, allowing proactive staffing.

These are not just efficiency metrics. They are measures of compassion. When patients move smoothly through the system, anxiety decreases, outcomes improve, and healthcare workers experience less moral distress.

Educating and Communicating Better: The Osler AI Example

Another transformative role for AI lies in how we educate and communicate. Traditional medical learning has always been limited by time, geography, and access to mentors. Osler AI, a Canadian innovation in digital medical education, is changing that.

Osler uses AI to simulate clinical cases, provide instant feedback, and tailor learning to each user's strengths and weaknesses. A trainee managing a simulated sepsis case receives real-time coaching: what to prioritize, when to escalate, how to communicate with patients and families. The AI not only tests knowledge but improves reasoning and communication under pressure.

Hospitals are beginning to adapt similar models for onboarding and team communication. Imagine a virtual assistant that briefs you before rounds, summarizes patient updates, or helps translate complex information into plain language for families. These tools don't just make us smarter, but more connected and consistent.

The future of AI in healthcare isn't just diagnostics or data. It's dialogue. Systems like Osler AI remind us that every algorithm, at its best, should strengthen human connection rather than replace it.

Augmenting Clinicians: Not Replacing Them

Despite the headlines, AI's greatest promise is not automation, but liberation. By taking over repetitive cognitive and clerical tasks, it gives clinicians back the time and focus they have lost. The most striking example is AI scribes. Across North America, these tools are already transforming practice. They listen to the clinical encounter, transcribe the conversation in real time, and generate a structured note that integrates directly into the electronic medical record.

Documentation has long been one of the biggest drivers of burnout. Physicians spend nearly half their workday on data entry. Early results from Canadian and U.S. pilots show that AI scribes can reduce documentation time by up to 60 percent and increase daily patient throughput by 15–20 percent.

The downstream effects are powerful. Clinicians report higher satisfaction, better eye contact with patients, and less after-hours charting. Finishing a shift with energy instead of exhaustion is not a trivial outcome. It is a wellness intervention. AI scribes are proof that technology can re-humanize care by removing the noise that once suffocated it.

Population Health: Seeing the Forest and the Trees

AI also allows us to look beyond the individual encounter and see the patterns shaping entire populations. Integrated data from primary care, pharmacies, and public health agencies can reveal early signals of crisis: rising blood pressure in one neighborhood, increased respiratory illness in another.

In British Columbia, predictive analytics have been used to anticipate opioid overdoses by geography, enabling pre-positioning of harm-reduction teams. Internationally, Singapore's Ministry of Health has deployed AI to forecast chronic-disease trends, allowing targeted prevention programs.

Population-level intelligence turns data into policy, helping systems act upstream rather than react downstream. For policymakers, this is how prevention becomes measurable and fundable.

Ethics, Equity, and Trust

For all its promise, AI raises profound ethical questions. Algorithms trained on biased datasets can reinforce inequities rather than dismantle them. Data privacy must be treated as a public trust, not a commodity.

Canadian provinces are beginning to address this through emerging frameworks for responsible AI in healthcare. Ontario Health and the Canadian Institutes of Health Research are developing national standards emphasizing transparency, explainability, and public engagement. Globally, the World Health Organization has called for "human oversight at every level" of AI-driven care. The principle is simple: technology should augment, not replace, human judgment.

Ethical AI must also be accessible AI. If only the privileged benefit from precision health, the digital divide will deepen health disparities. Policymakers must ensure that connectivity, affordability, and literacy accompany innovation.

The Human Opportunity

If these developments sound futuristic, they're not. They are already happening in academic centers, community hospitals, and start-ups across the world. What remains is alignment: leadership that connects innovation with purpose.

Technology alone will not fix healthcare, but technology guided by values might.

> AI cannot replicate empathy or intuition, but it can restore what clinicians and patients both crave: time.

Time to listen, time to think, time to heal. Used wisely, AI doesn't make medicine less human; it makes it more human.

Leadership and Policy Implications: The VIPA Framework in Action

Frameworks mean little until they are lived. The principles of Values, Integration, Pareto Focus, and Action are already shaping projects that prove what responsible AI can look like in the real world.

Mindstride – Human-Centered Mental-Health Technology

Mindstride was designed around values over fear. From day one, its creators asked, “How do we preserve dignity and privacy while using AI to help people feel better faster?” That question guided every decision, from encrypted journaling to transparent data policies.

Integration happened through co-design: clinicians, behavioral scientists, and software engineers built the tool together so that clinical insight informed every algorithm.

In line with the Pareto principle, Mindstride focused first on the 20 percent of interventions: movement reminders, brief journaling prompts, and social-connection nudges that drive most of the mental-health benefit. Rather than chase every metric, the team refined what worked.

Finally, action came through rapid piloting in Canadian workplaces. Outcomes were tracked in real time, feedback loops were short, and results (lower anxiety scores, higher engagement) guided the next version. Mindstride demonstrates that AI can scale compassion when built through VIPA.

Virtual Critical Care (VCC) – Technology Extending Expertise

VCC applies the same logic at a system level. Its values are clear: equitable access to ICU-level expertise no matter where a patient lives. Small hospitals in northern or rural regions deserve the same quality of monitoring and consultation as tertiary centers.

Integration links data science with frontline clinical workflow. Advanced analytics flag patients at risk of deterioration, while critical-care specialists connect virtually to guide local teams.

The Pareto focus keeps the project sustainable. VCC targets the few conditions and early-warning indicators that account for most ICU transfers, such as sepsis, respiratory failure, or post-operative decline.

Finally, VCC's Action is measured by results: fewer transfers, lower costs, shorter lengths of stay, and families kept closer to home. It shows that values-based innovation is not a slogan. It's an operational model.

Together, Mindstride and VCC illustrate what happens when the VIPA framework moves from concept to execution: AI becomes a bridge between technology and trust, efficiency and empathy, data and dignity.

Final Thoughts

From the wrist to the ward, from the home to the hospital, AI is reshaping healthcare's nervous system. It can predict crises before they happen, personalize prevention, and restore balance to systems that have long been overwhelmed.

The challenge now is to steer this transformation with integrity. Canada, with its integrated public system and strong academic networks, is uniquely positioned to lead a global model of ethical, efficient, and compassionate AI adoption.

If we embrace this moment, guided by our values, grounded in evidence, and unified in purpose, we can create a system that finally flows: one that is smart, sustainable, and profoundly human.

The future of healthcare is already here. Our task is to ensure it serves everyone.

Reflection

1. What future are we willing to build if we stop accepting the status quo as inevitable?
2. What is one courageous action you can take, from your current role, to help move healthcare from reaction to prevention?

Key Takeaways

- Technology should restore flow, and humanity.
- Ethical AI requires human-centered design and privacy protections.
- Predictive analytics can improve triage, prevention, and resources.

Conclusion
A Different Future Is Possible

This book was never just about habits. And it was never just about prevention. It's about changing the trajectory of healthcare itself.

After years in the ICU, I've seen the limits of a system built on reaction. We wait for disease... then mobilize everything to treat it. And while that system saves lives, it's overwhelmed, expensive, and, too often, too late. What became clear to me is this:

We don't have a healthcare system.

We have a sick-care system.

And if we want better outcomes, we can't just work harder within it. We have to reimagine it. That's where this book comes in.

Yes, we talked about prevention. Yes, we talked about the PRESS method (Purpose, Restoration, Eating, Strength, and Social connection). Because those are the foundations of health. But we also talked about something just as important:

How we redesign the system around those principles.

Through frameworks like VIPA (Values, Integrative thinking, Pareto focus, and Action), we start to see what real change looks like. Not theory. Not talk. But execution.

We've already started to see what's possible. Through initiatives like Black Med Collective, we've built community and created space for voices that were missing. Through Lionheart, we've brought together clinicians, innovators, and entrepreneurs to think differently about healthcare. Through **Mindstride**, we've begun to integrate prevention, mental health, and primary care, leveraging virtual care to improve access and continuity.

We've explored new models, private-public partnerships, hybrid care, proactive assessments, all designed around one idea:

Meet people earlier. Help them stay well. Reduce the need for crisis care.

This is what healthcare reform actually looks like. Not one big policy change, but thousands of small, aligned shifts:

- Clinicians thinking upstream
- Systems prioritizing prevention
- Technology improving access, not adding complexity
- Communities taking ownership of their health

And here's the part that gives me the most hope:

This isn't a distant future. It's already happening.

We have the tools, the knowledge, and the people. What we need now is the willingness to think differently and the courage to act.

And that future starts with both individual action and system leadership. Yes, you taking control of your health matters.

But so does:

- How we design clinics
- How we train clinicians
- How we fund care
- How we build communities

This is your invitation.

To take ownership of your health.

To challenge the status quo.

To think bigger than the current system.

Because change doesn't come from waiting. It comes from people who are willing to do things differently.

So, start simple. Pick your 1–2 highest-impact actions using the PRESS method. Apply the Pareto principle.

Focus on what moves the needle.

But don't stop there. Ask better questions. Push for better systems. Build, support, and advocate for new models of care. Because if we get this right, we don't just help individuals live better. We transform healthcare.

Let's build a future where:

- Prevention is the foundation
- Access is seamless
- Care is proactive
- And fewer people ever need to meet me in the ICU

That future is possible.

And it starts now.

References

Berwick, D. M., Nolan, T. W., & Whittington, J. (2008). The Triple Aim: Care, health, and cost. *Health Affairs, 27*(3), 759-769.

Bodenheimer, T., & Sinsky, C. (2014). From Triple to Quadruple Aim: Care of the patient requires care of the provider. *Annals of Family Medicine, 12*(6), 573-576.

Canadian Institute for Health Information. (2024). *National Health Expenditure Trends*. CIHI.

Canadian Institute for Health Information. (2024). *Wait Times for Priority Procedures in Canada*. CIHI.

Davenport, T., & Kalakota, R. (2019). The potential for artificial intelligence in healthcare. *Future Healthcare Journal, 6*(2), 94-98.

Detering, K. M., Hancock, A. D., Reade, M. C., & Silvester, W. (2010). The impact of advance care planning on end-of-life care in elderly patients: Randomised controlled trial. *BMJ, 340*, c1345.

Edmondson, A. C. (2018). *The Fearless Organization: Creating Psychological Safety in the Workplace for Learning, Innovation, and Growth*. Wiley.

Greenhalgh, T., Robert, G., Macfarlane, F., Bate, P., & Kyriakidou, O. (2004). Diffusion of innovations in service organizations: Systematic review and recommendations. *The Milbank Quarterly, 82*(4), 581-629.

Holt-Lunstad, J., Smith, T. B., & Layton, J. B. (2010). Social relationships and mortality risk: A meta-analytic review. *PLOS Medicine, 7*(7), e1000316.

Institute of Medicine. (2001). *Crossing the Quality Chasm: A New Health System for the 21st Century*. National Academies Press.

Kahneman, D. (2011). *Thinking, Fast and Slow*. Farrar, Straus and Giroux.

Kotter, J. P. (2012). *Leading Change*. Harvard Business Review Press.

Marteau, T. M., Ogilvie, D., Roland, M., Suhrcke, M., & Kelly, M. P. (2011). Judging nudging: Can nudging improve population health? *BMJ, 342*, d228.

National Academies of Sciences, Engineering, and Medicine. (2019). *Taking Action Against Clinician Burnout: A Systems Approach to Professional Well-Being*. National Academies Press.

OECD. (2017). *Tackling Wasteful Spending on Health*. OECD Publishing.

OECD. (2023). *Health at a Glance 2023: OECD Indicators*. OECD Publishing.

Porter, M. E., & Teisberg, E. O. (2006). *Redefining Health Care: Creating Value-Based Competition on Results*. Harvard Business School Press.

Rajkomar, A., Dean, J., & Kohane, I. (2019). Machine learning in medicine. *New England Journal of Medicine, 380*(14), 1347-1358.

Starfield, B., Shi, L., & Macinko, J. (2005). Contribution of primary care to health systems and health. *The Milbank Quarterly, 83*(3), 457-502.

Stacey, D., Legare, F., Lewis, K., Barry, M. J., Bennett, C. L., Eden, K. B., Holmes-Rovner, M., Llewellyn-Thomas, H., Lyddiatt, A., Thomson, R., & Trevena, L. (2017). Decision aids for people facing health treatment or screening decisions. *Cochrane Database of Systematic Reviews*, CD001431.

Thaler, R. H., & Sunstein, C. R. (2008). *Nudge: Improving Decisions About Health, Wealth, and Happiness*. Yale University Press.

Topol, E. (2019). *Deep Medicine: How Artificial Intelligence Can Make Healthcare Human Again*. Basic Books.

World Health Organization. (2018). *Declaration of Astana*. WHO.

World Health Organization. (2021). *Ethics and Governance of Artificial Intelligence for Health: WHO Guidance*. WHO.

World Health Organization. (2022). *Global Strategy on Digital Health 2020-2025*. WHO.

About the Author

Dr. Kwadwo Kyeremanteng is an intensive care physician, healthcare leader, and advocate for healthy living. Passionate about preventing illness rather than treating it, Dr. Kyeremanteng promotes a holistic approach to wellness through nutrition, fitness, stress management, and community engagement. He is the founder of Gyata Nutrition and hosts the Prevention Over Prescription podcast, sharing insights and strategies to inspire healthier lifestyles. Dedicated to innovation in healthcare, he co-founded Lionheart Innovation and co-founded the non-profit organizations Bridges Over Barriers and the Black Medical Collective. Dr. Kyeremanteng resides with his family, dedicated to leading by example in all aspects of life.

Instagram: @kwadcast

LinkedIn: https://www.linkedin.com/in/kwadwo-kyeremanteng/

Website: https://drkwadwo.ca/

Email: kwadcast99@gmail.com

thank you

Thank you for reading my book!

Thank you for taking this journey with me. Writing this book and sharing these insights has been deeply rewarding, and I hope it inspires you to take action. Remember, you are not alone in this process. There's a community of like-minded individuals—friends, family, and even people you've never met—who are on this journey with you. Lean on them, share your wins, and help each other grow.

One thing I've learned through my years in medicine and wellness is this: small, consistent actions can lead to profound transformations. Start today, stay consistent, and trust that your effort will pay off.

To your health and happiness,
Dr. Kwadwo Kyeremanteng

MY GIFT TO YOU

I am so glad you're here!

As my Gift to you, get FREE Access to resources and other bonus content by scanning the QR Code below or visiting drkwadwo.ca